GUT LOGIC

A Scientific Approach to Improving Your Gut Microbiome

Graham C. Mackenzie Ph.C.
with Dragana Skokovic-Sunjic RPh BScPhm NCMP
& Lindsay Dixon RPh BScPhm

Copyright © 2023 by Ultimate Publishing House

GUT LOGIC
The Power of the Microbiome to Transform Your Health

By: Graham C. Mackenzie PH.C.

All rights reserved as this book may not be reproduced in whole or in part, by any means, without written consent of the publisher.

For permission requests, write to the publisher, addressed

"Attention: Permissions Coordinator" at the address below:

THE ULTIMATE PUBLISHING HOUSE (UPH)
Canadian Office: 205 Glen Shields Avenue
Toronto, Ontario,
Canada L4K 2B0
Telephone: 647-883-1758

www.GutLogicBook.com

www.ultimatepublishinghouse.com
E-mail: info@ultimatepublishinghouse.com

Quantity discounts are available on bulk purchases of this book for reselling, educational purposes, subscription incentives, gifts, sponsorship, or fundraising. Unique books or book excerpts can also be fashioned to suit special needs such as private labeling with your logo on the cover and a message from or a message printed on the second page of the book.

For more information, please contact our Special Sales Department at Ultimate Publishing House. Orders for college textbook or course adoption use.

Please contact Ultimate Publishing House Tel: 647-883-1758

GUT LOGIC
The Power of the Microbiome to Transform Your Health
By: Graham C. Mackenzie PH.C.

ISBN: 979-8-9882088-9-1

Table Of Contents

Introduction
(Contribution by Dragana Skokovic-Sunjic). 5

Chapter 1: The Logic about our Gut 15

Chapter 2: Exploring Upper Respiratory
Tract Infections (URTI's). 29

Chapter 3: Understanding Diarrhea. 33

Chapter 4: Insight into Irritable Bowel Syndrome (IBS) 37

Chapter 5: Nurturing Mental Health 41

Chapter 6: Navigating Bacterial Vaginosis and
Vulvovaginal Candidiasis (Yeast Infection) 47

Chapter 7: Unveiling Urinary Tract Infections (UTI's) . 53

Chapter 8: Cervical Cancer Awareness. 57

Chapter 9: Strategies for Effective Weight Loss 59

Chapter 10: Managing Cholesterol Levels 63

Chapter 11: Tackling Eczema. 67

Chapter 12: Exploring the World of Fermented Foods
and Prebiotics 71

Introduction

(Dragana Skokovic-Sunjic contribution)

Probiotics. An interesting word—the word that we did not know very much about some twenty years ago. We did not even use it that frequently, and now probiotics are everywhere. It's in your food, in your supplements, in your shampoo, and in your skin cream.

The question is, what are probiotics? Is there a definition or a rule that we must use to call something probiotic, and what is the big fuss about? Let's try to look back at the beginning.

Humans have massive amounts and vast quantities of living and dying bacteria in their gut. Bacteria are primarily in our gut, but they can be found everywhere, on our skin, in our mouth, and elsewhere. Everywhere in and on our body, we have these communities of hopefully mostly good bugs, living, thriving, dying off, and renewing their colonies. Why do we have them? They support our health; they break down foods we cannot digest and produce by-products that support our overall health. They regulate many different processes in our body, not only in our gut but for our immune system and overall health.

So, the idea is to keep those communities of live bacteria, our microbiome, happy, healthy, and functioning well. We do this by various means: a good lifestyle, great food choices, and avoiding harmful influences such as different medications, antibiotics, excessive alcohol, etc.

However, there is sometimes a possibility or opportunity to use a probiotic, another live bacterium, to support our gut microbiome and ensure things are working well.

That sounds straightforward: take some bacteria, and all will be well. Not so fast. In school, we learned that bacteria or microbes could be deadly. There are horrible infections caused by bacteria, and some life-threatening issues are caused by a simple microbe. Harmful bugs can take over and cause disease, leading to complications from which we can die. That is why we use antibiotics to kill that harmful bacteria and resolve the problem; again, very simple.

When we talk about bacteria being used as an intervention or as a therapy in the form of probiotics, we must tread very carefully. With events and discoveries of good microbes in fermented foods a century or more ago, we learned that homemade yogurts, kefir, or other fermented foods could provide live cultures. These living bacteria would support our health. Fast forward a hundred years, and we now have those live bacteria in different forms, such as capsules, sachets, tablets, and fortified drinks, in much higher amounts. How do we know whether these bacteria are going to be helpful or not? How do we know if these bacteria will not cause an infection or worsen our problems?

Regulations exist across the globe, and different countries have their own set of rules: what can be called probiotics, how do we market the probiotics, how do we package and label them, and how do we sell them? Globally, there exists a definition of probiotics. It was first introduced in 2001 by WHO/FAO. That was the first time we had groups of scientists, including the leading Canadian researcher, Dr. Gregor Reid, develop a proper definition. At the time, the probiotic was defined as "live microorganisms that, when administered in adequate amounts, confer a health benefit on the host".[1]

That definition was updated in 2015 with some small grammar changes. Right now, that definition reads that a probiotic is "live microorganisms that, when administered in adequate amounts, confer a health benefit on the host."[2]

Now that we have a definition of probiotics, your local grocery store, pharmacy, and health food store are teeming with hundreds of probiotic products. That means they all must be working, correct?

How do we know what happens when we take these capsules containing 10–15 different bacteria while sleeping and waiting to be woken up to start working in our gut? How do we know they will do well, perform a good task, and not wreak havoc in our gut? Is there a difference between products, and why do we have so many different products and so many different probiotics?

To better understand what happens when we take a probiotic, let's imagine our body is a house. Imagine everything is working fine in your home—electricity, plumbing—and it is a lovely and cozy house. Occasionally, you might get guests coming through, and they make you feel good. You have a party, have fun, and then the guests leave. You keep great memories and feel good for some time after. Rarely do those party people stay in your house forever. So those people who came for the party would be probiotics or fermented foods you have on occasion. They support your gut microbiome. They do not stay forever, and they do not colonize the gut. That is a widespread belief that comes to mind when talking about the gut microbiome and probiotics—probiotics do not stay in your gut forever. Probiotics rarely colonize the gut.

Let's say something breaks in your house. For example, your faucet is broken, and there is water spraying everywhere. It is flooding your kitchen. There is a problem, and you need to get someone to fix it. Do you go to your door and call everybody to come in and help you, or do you dial your trusted plumber to fix it? Do you call your electrician to fix your plumbing or your grandmother to replace your facet? No, you do not.

That means you are selecting a probiotic or bacteria that will be helpful for your issues and one that has the evidence to support it. Like your plumber having his certificate or proof, he knows what he is doing.

If you have a problem that you think probiotics can fix, you will select one with supporting evidence. Not all probiotics will be the same, and not all bacterial strains will do the same job. Same as the people around you. Your grandma might not be the one to fix your faucet. She is a lovely grandma, but not helpful for your particular problem.

When you are fixing something, you select the appropriate means to do it.

Let's go back to your plumbing problem. You called the expert, your trusted plumber. Maybe he comes in alone or with an assistant. And they will fix your issue in 10–15 minutes. Do you then call 15 or 20 plumbers to come in together? Or do you call a few electricians just in case, and your grandma's bridge club members, to come all together? Because the more, the merrier.

It would not end well. If there are more people crowding in your kitchen who think they know what they are doing, it is going to be a big mess, maybe even a fight. The good plumber will be blocked off, and he will have no room to move and be very upset with the situation.

This is akin to taking a probiotic product with lots of different strains. And as many as possible billions of bacteria are in it.

A similar way of thinking when it comes to probiotics is that people often select products with as many strains as possible or as many CFU (colony-forming units) as possible, thinking it will provide more benefit.

It is not going to end well unless there is proof. You may genuinely need five plumbers to fix your problem. But it would be best if you found out what the evidence is, what other people with the same problem used, and how they fixed it. Or, if you are not a fan of reading the published studies, which can be confusing, you will ask your healthcare provider, physician, pharmacist, or dietitian for help.

Many healthcare professionals have had the same questions you have about probiotics over the last few decades. Most of us were amazed by the published research and evidence growing exponentially year after year, looking at the potential for probiotics as an intervention. However, most of us were confused with the question: How do I know what probiotics to recommend? This particular study is telling me I should be recommending this complicated-sounding strain of Lactobacillus rhamnosus with a series of letters and numbers behind it. If I gave this name to my patient, would they know what product to buy?

It would be the same as recommending a plumber; if you do not provide his name and phone number, that will not be a helpful recommendation.

Years ago, we started sorting through the published evidence, finding what particular strain or set combination of strains performed well in the study, helping actual patients, not mice or rats, improve their health in a meaningful way. The next step was finding a product available in Canada or the US with the same strain or combination and connecting the dots to help figure out what to recommend. That is why we came up with the Clinical Guide to Probiotic Products, with Canadian and US issues published separately, as product names and offerings might differ. Year after year, this resource had to be updated annually because of a few things: evidence is growing each year, product names can change, the company might decide to change the strains in the products, or the quantity can change.[3]

These are things we try to keep up to date and issue new guides year after year.

Going back to our house issues: just as a conclusion Yes, it would be best if you got an expert for your house problem. You need to know about his reputation (evidence).

Another question is: Does that plumber need to move in with us after fixing our plumbing issue? I do not think so; after he is done, he will leave. If the problem happens again, you can call the same expert again. As with a good probiotic, it will help you fix the problem and then go.

If you keep getting the same problem frequently, even after fixing it, maybe you need a thorough house inspection to discover the underlying problem—an investigation with your physician.

There are a few other interesting points I like to address when it comes to probiotics:

Select a specific strain for your particular problem.

Select the amount that is proven to work; do not go with the "the more, the merrier" idea.

Most of us do not need to take probiotics forever unless we have a chronic condition and our healthcare provider recommends it.

A wrong belief exists that refrigerated probiotics are better than those at room temperature. It all depends on the strain. Some strains are resilient and resistant to the influence of oxygen, light, and temperature and stay viable after exposure; other strains are very fragile and need to be protected, kept in dark bottles, specific formulations, and refrigerated to prolong their viability.

You do not need to get your gut tested to see what is missing. Each of us has a different blend and composition of the gut microbiome. Each of us has a different house; they might look similar from the outside, but inside, we are very different:

furniture, decoration, scent, souvenirs, and our living spaces are filled with our unique things. Even if you move from one space to another, the inside of your home will be very similar to your old house because we like to keep things the same.

As newborns, we start collecting messages from our mother's gut in utero, picking up bacteria as soon as we are born from our mothers, environment, caregivers, and the food we eat. That bacterium quite rapidly starts setting up in our gut. By age 3 or 5, we all have our own unique blend of gut bacteria; more or less, we will keep it fairly consistent throughout life. The lifestyle will influence the composition from time to time.

Like when we move into a new house, we quickly get the furnishings. Over the years, we might update some furnishings.

Testing the gut microbiome and getting recommendations based on the test is similar to attempts to furnish all our homes the same. It will not work.

Testing of the microbiome exists, and it is used for research purposes. We can still learn a lot about that. There are substantial global initiatives to gather as much information about gut microbiome compositions as possible. For now, there is no good reason to pay for the test.

Chapter 1

THE LOGIC ABOUT OUR GUT

The topic of probiotics and their effects when given to healthy or diseased individuals is, to say the least, complicated. One thing is certain: the digestive tracts of our bodies contain hundreds of strains of healthy bacteria, amounting to trillions of microorganisms that do exert some benefits to our health as we age. The potential of this reach is staggering. From the digestion of food to the creation of vitamins and nutrients, mood, immune function, sleep quality, and overall integrity of our bodies, probiotics are an asset that we haven't been able to scratch the surface of in their effect. It is important to note here that the microbiome, which represents the normal flora of bacteria in our body, is not just restricted to the gut. Although most research is done on the gut microbiome, the entire body is involved with its own microbiome in various compartments. The skin is alive with all types of organisms, not just bacteria. Various areas of the body harbour different communities of bacteria. Males and females are also different. Those living in different climates, different ages, and using different cleaning products and lifestyle choices all create a microbiome on the skin as individuals as you are. The flora of the mouth is different from the large and small bowels. The flora involved with the respiratory system and urogenital system are also unique on their own. Each system has an invaluable contribution to all aspects of your health, from your susceptibility to infection to your reproductive health, your mood, and so much more.[4]

What makes probiotics so complicated? Can't we just throw a few strains in a capsule and give that daily to repopulate the gut with "healthy bacteria" that it not only should have anyway but also has shown to have some health effects? Isn't it similar to the concept of keeping healthy grass growing on your lawn to prevent weeds from taking over? It turns out that the healthy flora of the gut is so complicated that just throwing at the gut probiotics isn't really the answer.

In fact, some people simply don't respond the same way as others to probiotics. Some retain them, and some don't. Some GI systems accept them, or maybe more correctly, some probiotics accept some GI systems, and others do not.

Sometimes it becomes easier to take the flora from a healthy person and transplant it into an unhealthy GI than to try to figure out what to give orally. Not the most practical or desired route for the patient. One thing is clear: without healthy flora, we lack optimal GI health. And without optimal GI health, our bodies are not working at peak performance. Just to give you some sense of how important this is, consider the flora of a mouse that is overweight transplanted into that of a lean mouse, and the lean mouse gains weight. Hopefully, this grabs your attention. But what should also grab your attention is that this book is based on the absolute best evidence to date. With all well-designed scientific studies, there are responders and non-responders. My hope is that what works, as shown by science, works for you. From personal clinical experience, I can attest to the response probiotics can give you when the right ones are taken in the right amounts.

What causes the flora to become unbalanced and in need of repair in the first place? Well, there are many causes. Being on an antibiotic for any length of time can obviously alter this distribution. Infections by unfriendly agents can also do this. Anything that affects the immune system, including certain medications and stress, can also affect the flora of your gut. Inflammation, the cause of many health issues, can also affect the gut flora and function. To know who can be best helped by probiotics, we need to follow the best evidence of what has been studied to date.

Mentioned earlier in the book is the work of one of its contributors, Dragana Skokovic-Sunjic, a clinical pharmacist who has authored "Clinical Guide to Probiotic Products Available in Canada and the US." This is a one-of-a kind reference that is reflected online at AEProbio.com. The reason why this site is so valued, in my opinion, is because it does something that most other references do not. Dragana and her colleagues give the pedestrian reader the exact commercial product that corresponds to the strain or strains that have evidence of working. As I have explained to many health professionals and in this book, simply telling someone probiotics work or don't work for a medical condition means nothing without the actual product referenced as well. Most people will hunt forever for that product unless given the name. Just like when a doctor calls in a prescription, they tell me what drug they want and what dose. Probiotics are no different. It is for this reason that I reference actual brand names in some of the sections going forward when they are available and there is evidence for them. As a disclaimer, I have not reached out to give these companies a heads-up. I am mentioning their product and am not and will not accept anything in the way of a donation or educational grant from them for mentioning their product. This book is for you. My first goal is to get the information out to you to improve your health.

It's also important to know what level of evidence I am referencing when I recommend a product to use for a given medical condition, which should always be done in conjunction with your healthcare providers, like your prescribers and your pharmacists. AEProbio uses three levels of evidence. Collecting evidence in the OTC and supplement sections of the pharmacy is always difficult because not many companies want to foot the bill for something another company can take and sell as their own, but we have a respectable amount of evidence that is growing for probiotics. My previous book, Healthy Logic, helps to explain what makes a good study and what makes a bad study.

Level I Evidence: Evidence obtained from at least one appropriately designed trial (e.g., randomization of subjects given the active agent or placebo, blinding of experimenters to who is receiving the active agent or placebo, and appropriate population comparisons) with a power calculation for the outcomes of interest. This means the study is strong enough to conclude what it proposes (the highest level of evidence).

Level II evidence is obtained from well-designed placebo-controlled trials without randomization; evidence obtained from randomized trials does not satisfy all criteria listed in Level I. Evidence obtained from well-designed cohort or case-control analytic studies, preferably from more than one centre or research group, Evidence obtained from multiple time series with or without the intervention Dramatic results in uncontrolled trials might also be regarded as this type of evidence.

Level III Evidence: Opinions of respected authorities, based on clinical experience, descriptive studies, or reports of expert committees.

As you can see, the strength of the levels of evidence decreases as you go down this list from level I to level III. I will be referring to these levels when I give recommendations, so you'll know the strength of the recommendation.

You should know who this recommendation of probiotics is for. It may surprise you to know that supplementing with probiotics isn't for everyone. Most people who are relatively healthy and symptom-free of bothersome issues really aren't going to benefit much from probiotics. There really is very little evidence to support taking random probiotics or even targeted probiotics, for that matter, for long-term health outcomes. This needs to be laid out right out of the gate. You should be wary of recommendations for supplements that don't have an end date or are without a scientific basis unless your physician deems it necessary. Even with an existing condition, probiotics are meant to be used within a defined period, as we will see for the most part. If you fall within the boundaries laid out for each reason for taking a probiotic (which is almost everyone at some point in their life), then this book is your reference. You should always strive for better health; you just need to know where your money is best spent over your entire lifetime to age in a healthy manner. Quite often, probiotics are effective when taken until they work, and continued use may not really be warranted.

The picture of life with these guidelines not only means better gut health but also better overall health, less infection, fewer disease symptoms, less medication, and more awareness of your overall health when you are able to choose what you eat. Barriers to this becoming a reality are many. Not the least of which is the affordability of healthy recommended food. Not just financially, but the food environment you live in may simply not lend itself to healthy choices based on a busy lifestyle. Telling people what they should eat and how they should live is one of the toughest things a healthcare professional can do when their life situation is taken into account. The effect stress has on your gut is well established. Telling someone to reduce stress is a nice goal to shoot for, but we aren't expecting them to up and leave their job or bad relationship tomorrow. The goal is to live as long as possible, upright, moving, and enjoying your life. When all evidence is taken into account, I believe probiotics can play a role in that when carefully and thoughtfully chosen at various points in your life.

The key that makes these recommendations unique is that they lay out the science of various medical issues one by one. They don't paint all probiotics and medical conditions with one brush. It is important to realize that the recommendation of a specific probiotic is as important as a physician writing for a specific antibiotic and dose for the particular infection that has stricken you. You need the recommendation right down to the ultra-specific probiotic needed and its dose. Otherwise, you are just taking a "probiotic" for the sake of taking one. This book uses the most up-to-date evidence that tells us what works with probiotics and what doesn't. As a consumer, you may be left out in the cold, not knowing what brand of probiotic has the exact strains you need for a given ailment. This will be laid out for you. Up until now, you may have been "recommended" probiotics by a well-meaning health professional, but now you have the reason why I am recommending very specific brands. That is why this time will be different.

Although we may still lack the full reason why a certain strain or multitude of strains improve a condition or prevent one from occurring, we do know one thing: if a well-designed study with the power to conclude that a given probiotic works for a given medical issue decides that it works, then we recommend it. Each section will outline what you should use and what else you should do to maximize the effect of normal flora. The goal is to let you live your life as much as possible, but be mindful of the simple steps you can take to effect change in your health.

The critical component is to match your health concerns with the correct brand of probiotics and prebiotics. Extra information can be found as outlined at AEProbio.com, a wonderful reference to check in on. Above all, seek out someone in your healthcare circle who is knowledgeable about probiotics and prebiotics. This book will give you a good foundation, but for day-to-day advice on this growing topic, you need a go-to person that can support you. Maybe that person is your pharmacist, maybe a dietician, or maybe your doctor. Either way, it helps to have a person to bounce things off of.

WHAT MAKES A GUT UNHEALTHY?

In fact, there is much more to a healthy gut than just healthy flora. It would be a disservice to merely say, Take probiotics and be done with it. We know there is so much more to our health than making a specific recommendation and expecting results. The human body is so much more complicated than that. Let's look at some of the things we need to be mindful of to be sure a dose of probiotics does what science says it should do.

MEDICATIONS

We should get this one out of the way right out of the gate. In modern medicine, any medical doctrine relies on one major factor: the risk-benefit ratio. We accept the potential for side effects, intensity, and risk to our health that medications give; we just accept that the reason we are taking a given medication and the potential benefit outweigh that risk. It's basically how I do my job as a pharmacist. Now, before you get on the big pharma bandwagon, we should also accept that most of what we do in life follows the same principle. From putting our feet on the floor when we get out of bed in the morning to driving a car to work, walking into work and doing our job, eating a mealtime, or going on a trip, Most of the time, the practice is subconscious and automatic from experience. We just do what we do in life without much thought, knowing that life can change at the drop of a hat from something going wrong.

This brings us to medications that we often take daily. Anti-inflammatory drugs (NSAIDS) are near the top of the list of medications that can have incredible damaging effects on the gut, especially when taken regularly. The damage can be so severe that even probiotics would be useless to undo the adverse effects. Not just the direct irritant effect of NSAIDS but their downstream effect, whereby they reduce prostaglandins, which naturally protect the lining of our digestive system against damage, NSAIDS have far-reaching adverse effect potential on our gut.

Antibiotics, because of the adverse effect they have on the normal flora of the gut, can be damaging, especially when overused. A single dose of a strong antibiotic like clindamycin or ciprofloxacin can result in months of self-repair by the gut to get back to normal. Hidden sources of antibiotics, like meat, can also affect the microbiome. Other medications that change our normal bacteria in the gut include a certain medication used for GI problems. Proton pump inhibitors (PPI's) effectively reduce acid in the stomach and can allow more offending agents to survive the passage into the small and large intestines. Regular antacids also run this risk.

The bone-builder bisphosphonate family, like alendronate and risedronate, can be particularly corrosive to the upper GI tract, which is why we give specific directions to stay upright for at least an hour after taking them. Potassium can cause direct damage to the entire GI tract. It is important to not take it on an empty stomach, and it is also helpful to take it with a full glass of water to help prevent this. Also important is the prevention of constipation, including constipating medications. While taking potassium supplementation, make sure it isn't in contact with any part of the digestive system for any period.

Oral contraceptives can also have a detrimental effect on the gut and have been implicated in causing inflammatory bowel disease. These drugs have a close relationship with the intestinal flora, to the point that there is potential for failure of the birth control effect when taken with antibiotics. Certain antidepressants like sertraline and other types of medications like carbamazepine, metformin, and lithium, as well as antipsychotic medications like olanzapine, risperidone, quetiapine, and in particular, clozapine, can all cause damage to the gut lining. Even without the drug, some excipients or non-drug ingredients found in medications can be harmful to the gut lining. Chemotherapeutic drugs are also quite damaging to the gut due to their prevention of the replication of cells with rapid turnover.

Of course, there are other things that can harm the gut that aren't medications. Alcohol is particularly damaging. There are many ways this can happen. For example, it is estimated that 30% of cancers in the mouth and throat are caused by drinking alcohol. Mucosal cells in the stomach that have a protective role are damaged by even a single heavy episode of alcohol ingestion. It relaxes the sphincter that keeps food from going back into the esophagus from the stomach. Intestinal cancers are also increased in those who regularly consume alcohol.

Various other mechanisms are at play when it comes to the health of our digestive system that we present to probiotics. Physical and emotional stress, general inflammation, and diet have a huge impact on the normal flora in your gut. The American Gut Project determined that the more plants a person eats, the more diverse the flora in the gut. We will discuss more of the beneficial effects of diet on your flora later. We know that the diet you consumed as a child has lifelong effects on your flora, which you carry through life. We are beginning to learn that the standard North American diet (excess fat and sugar) has detrimental effects on the flora, as does a lack of exercise.[5]

Coincidentally, omega-3 intake, which has an anti-inflammatory presence in our bodies, has been shown to have a favourable effect on the flora in our gut.[6]

This gives us a peek at what to expect from the state of our microbiome, even without trying to supplement with probiotics.

Chapter 2

EXPLORING UPPER RESPIRATORY TRACT INFECTIONS (URTI'S)

As mentioned, most of the studies that show what distribution we have of bacteria are involved with the gastrointestinal system, most commonly the small and large bowels. As we know, other tissues have their own normal flora. Let's look at the effect we can have on these tissues with probiotic ingestion. Respiratory tract infections result every year in countless days off work and added expense both publicly and privately, not to mention the mortality rate, especially in those more susceptible, like seniors, and those with pre-existing medical conditions that make these types of infections more dangerous, like asthma, COPD, diabetes, and autoimmune disorders.

The Cochrane Library is a resource that one typically goes to for well-researched studies on various medical topics. They are quite rigorous, so if they say something works or most likely works, you can believe them. Remember that it is imperative that any study on probiotics be specific to the exact strain and dose. In one review in 2022 of qualifying URTI studies, they looked at 24 studies that included almost 7,000 people of all ages, including infants, in multicenter locations all over the world. Most studies used lactobacillus plantarum HEAL9 and lactobacillus paracasei (8700:2 or N1115) and 109 to 1011 colony-forming units (CFU's) per day as a dose. They determined that there was a 24% reduction in those that got at least 1 URTI and a 43% reduction in those that got 3 URTI's. There was a 42% reduction in antibiotic use as well. They concluded that there is a benefit to using probiotics in preventing URTI's. Quite promising![7]

Another review was done in 2014 that looked at the incidence of ventilator-associated pneumonia (VAP), an infection that is common in ICUs when someone is ventilated for more than 48 hours. This review looked at 8 studies with over 1000 participants. The types of probiotics given were more wide-ranging (Lactobacillus casei rhamnosis, Lactobacillus plantarum, Synbiotic 2000FORTE, Eryphilus, and a combination of Bifidobacterium longum, Lactobacillus bulgaricus, and Streptococcus thermophilus). The results of this study were not as clear-cut, however. Although evidence suggested that using probiotics was associated with a reduction in the incidence of VAP, this was not clear across all studies. This demonstrates the complexity of utilizing probiotics for a given medical condition.[8]

Just to put into context the difficulty in interpreting the results of these experiments and applying them to real-life recommendations, the microbial species Bifidobacterium longum is a microbial species, but there are over 400 strains of this species. Different strains of the same species are all different and can have different biological activities.

Health Canada has given approval for this use with Level I evidence for the probiotic HMF Fit for School. A randomized, double-blinded, placebo-controlled study showed some efficacy with this product, which also includes a small amount of vitamin C (50 mg) and 1000 IU of vitamin D. It is important to note that lower respiratory tract infections were not affected by this product, however.[9]

Chapter 3

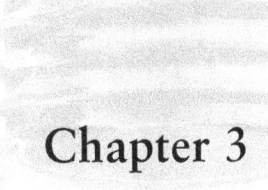

UNDERSTANDING DIARRHEA

What better use for a supplement that resides in the bowel and is used for digestion for people who have hypermotility issues? There is no shortage of legwork done here for you.

One meta-analysis in 2019 looked at 34 previous studies that pooled nearly 5,000 child patients. This study looked at patients who took not only probiotics but synbiotics as well. Synbiotics are a combination of probiotics and prebiotics, a non-digestible fibre that helps the host stimulate the growth and activity of potentially beneficial flora. There was a positive correlation between certain strains of probiotics, like Saccharomyces boulardii and Bifidobacterium, and the resolution of acute diarrhea. Lactobacillus was less effective. The duration of vomiting was also reduced, as was the potential for fever in these patients.[10]

Cochrane's also did a meta-analysis covering 33 studies involving 6300 children with antibiotic-associated diarrhea. This type of diarrhea is significant in its scope not only because it can result in interrupting the antibiotic dosing but also because it can lead to a more serious infection in the bowel due to the overgrowth of the wrong type of bug. The investigated probiotics here were Lactobacilli spp., Bifidobacterium spp., Streptococcus spp., or Saccharomyces boulardii, either alone or in combination. There was a benefit seen in treatments from 5 days to 12 weeks. The number of children needed to be treated (NNT) was 9, meaning that for every nine children treated, one showed benefit. This number might seem a bit high, but consider that most prescription drugs, in comparison, are often higher than this. It's more of a reflection of how many actually got the antibiotic-associated diarrhea in the control group in the first place. Not everyone will. But we treat everyone equally. Therefore, we need to treat extra people to get a benefit. The most beneficial of the probiotics was Lactobacillus rhamnosus or Saccharomyces boulardii in doses of 5–40 billion CFU daily.[11]

Speaking of dangerous bowel infections from antibiotic use, Clostridium difficile is one such infection that requires immediate treatment. In a Cochrane review of 39 trials and almost 10,000 patients, it was determined that probiotics conferred a 60% reduction in the risk of developing this infection while on antibiotics. When they isolated trials that involved high-risk patients, the risk reduction was even more pronounced at 70%. The most common side effects were abdominal cramping, nausea, fever, soft stools, and taste disturbance.[12]

Probiotics are often sought after for diarrhea of all types at all ages. Florastor and Florastor Max with a specific Saccharomyces boulardii are approved with Level I evidence for traveller diarrhea, antibiotic-associated diarrhea prevention, and C. difficile-associated diarrhea prevention through Health Canada. Also carrying the same weight of evidence and approval for prevention in C. difficile and travellers diarrhea is Bio-K+ Antibio Pro, as well as their two drinkable probiotics. If you're a fan of Culturelle, their Digestive Daily Probiotic

Chewables and Digestive Health Daily Probiotic Capsules have Level I evidence with Health Canada approval for the prevention of traveller diarrhea and antibiotic-associated diarrhea.

The Florastor Kids line can be used for ages 1–12 and has Level I evidence and Health Canada approval for the prevention of antibiotic-induced diarrhea and infectious diarrhea. This is a good time to mention that diarrhea, especially in kids and the elderly, can be serious, and you need to know when to seek medical help. It's not the scope of this book to cover this, but the main takeaway is that young kids, especially those under 1 year old, can become dehydrated quickly, and if you're in doubt, seek help. Your pharmacist is the most accessible healthcare professional here.

Chapter 4

INSIGHT INTO IRRITABLE BOWEL SYNDROME (IBS)

Irritable bowel syndrome, or IBS, is a common condition that is typically characterized by abdominal pain or discomfort and a change in bowel habits. Its presentation varies from person to person. Often, there is cramping or bloating, sharp pain, and distention. Some have mainly diarrhea; others have mainly constipation; and some alternate between the two. This condition can make the person afflicted miserable. Other symptoms can include migraine, anxiety, depression, chronic pelvic pain, and fibromyalgia. It is important to realize that any condition that you are treating over-the-counter for longer than a week or two (certainly a month) warrants bringing in your primary care provider to get their input. Treating IBS solely with probiotics for longer than a month is a signal from your body that even though you may feel better with probiotics, you may need some extra help in the form of medication.

Much work has been done to pin down the best recommendations for probiotics in IBS. To understand the immense task of finding an evidence-based approach to probiotics, the best analogy is to say we know probiotics help; we just need the best product specifically. For example, if you walked into a pharmacy and someone said one of the bottles on the dispensary shelf helped them and you knew nothing of medication, you might take away the opinion that any bottle would help with their blood pressure or any medical condition for that matter. Perhaps if you had diabetes, you would think any bottle on these magical shelves would also help you. In a way, this is where probiotics leave us. We know there is a benefit lying out there for probiotics; we just need to sift through the many different possibilities of which probiotic, what combination or individual one, and what strength will work for a given medical condition. To compound this, a given strain of probiotic may not be genetically the same as another bottler of the same probiotic. This strain-specificity discrepancy can mean different biologic activity.

This brings us to the opportunity to reinforce that probiotics may not bring us 100% relief, and we may need more help from other medications. For example, our DNA is capable of adapting over the long term to changing conditions, but when we compare the change in our intake of food over just the last 10,000 years to the snail's pace that our DNA struggles to adapt and change to, it's no wonder we have digestive problems that develop beyond the scope of probiotics. There is still hope, though, as we will now see from recent scientific studies on probiotics. Based on one meta-analysis, it appears that you will have better luck with a multistrain product (4–7 strains) with up to 10 billion CFU's per dose.[13]

Both lactobacillus and bifidobacterial have shown positive effects with a low incidence of adverse effects in over 80 trials with more than 10,000 patients.[14,15]

Commercially available products that have been tested for IBS are in high demand. IBS is not uncommon and can be debilitating for those who have it. Align and Align chewables, Bio-K+ IBS Pro, Digestive Care 10 Billion Daily Probiotic,

Purica Probiotic Intensive GI, and Ultra Flora Intensive Care are all health Canada-approved with Level I evidence for IBS for adults. Level II evidence with the same approval can be found with Biomed Bacillus Coagulans and HMF Metabolic.

For the pediatric population, Florastor Kids and Visbiome are approved by Health Canada for IBS in this population with Level I evidence.

Chapter 5

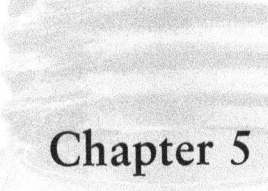

NURTURING MENTAL HEALTH

You may ask how the GI system could possibly have any effect on our mood, sleep, and mental wellbeing. It has been known for quite some time that the vast majority (perhaps as high as 95% of the total body serotonin) is provided by the gut. Serotonin plays a major role in mood, emotions, happiness, sleep, and pain. Also known is the gut-brain axis, a two-way communication between the gut and the central nervous system. Inflammation of this pathway by dysbiosis (a disruption in the microbiotic homeostasis) can change the amount of serotonin and dopamine released through this system. Not only does the integrity of the gut microbiome influence the serotonin we make, but now we know that drugs like antidepressants that target serotonin can have a major effect on our microbiome. The integrity of the barrier between the circulatory system and the brain, the gut, and the bloodstream become affected, as do the levels of proinflammatory mediators found in the blood. All contribute to a change in depressive symptoms.

A concept that is often overused is that of "leaky gut." Quite often, this term is thrown at a patient with chronic medical conditions as an explanation for why they are sick. Strictly speaking, leaky gut is often coined as a situation where there is increased intestinal permeability that allows larger molecules and microorganisms to be absorbed through the wall of the gut. The widely distributed theory is that this results in an inflammatory response in the body. Mention this to your doctor, and you may get a blank stare. That is because although the symptom of leaky gut is recognized, the downstream effect of what it does clinically is not really proven. My main reason for mentioning it here is the warning that although science is in agreement on what can damage the gut lining, leaky gut is a symptom and not a disease, and while there are some disease states like celiac, crohn's, irritable bowel, and even diabetes where increased intestinal permeability is not uncommon, the jury is still out on how much you should open your wallet to correct this problem to reverse or prevent autoimmune disease and chronic fatigue.

The contributing factors for "general public" leaky gut are stress and a bad diet, along with all of the other things we lay out in this book that contribute to an unhealthy gut lining. Depression would be one of the claimed effects of a leaky gut. Again, not backed by science. Again, leaky gut can be a sign of gut damage, and that could conceivably mean the serotonin or gut-brain axis might have issues with it, but it isn't a forgone conclusion.

One thing that is supported, however, is the existence of the gut-brain axis, which has a strong role in regulating stress-related responses. Moreover, gut microbiota have emerged as a critical component affecting signalling in those pathways. Conversely, stress can affect the makeup of our microbes in the gut. The gut-brain axis is a bi-directional connection between the gut and brain. They are connected by the prominent vegus nerve, and this serves as their communication line. Aside from this direct route, there are chemical messengers, hormones, and neurotransmitters that all help to create timely communication. The importance of the gut is reflected in the fact that many of the key molecules at play here are made there, including GABA, dopamine, and serotonin.

In relation to probiotic therapy and mood, conclusions are like in other medical applications with probiotics: although more studies are needed, current evidence shows that probiotics can have a beneficial effect on mood and depression. It has been found that when gut microtiota is altered experimentally, stress responsiveness and anxiety behaviour change. Above all, remember that mood disorders are nothing to mess around with, and it's important to not substitute these recommendations for standard therapy that your physician feels is recommended for you. By all means, rely on these recommendations as an add-on to your existing therapy.

In a review article published in 2020, a total of 10 trials were included, which included nearly 700 patients with depression combined with an anxiety component. Often, anxiety and depression symptoms go hand in hand, but not always. All patients in this review were 16 or older.[16]

Effects of Probiotics on Depressive or Anxiety Variables in Healthy Participants Under Stress Conditions or With a Depressive or Anxiety Diagnosis: A Meta-Analysis of Randomized Controlled Trials

It looked at studies no older than 5 years old. It found that probiotics were better at treating depression symptoms than anxiety. As well, probiotics were better at treating patients with anxiety and depression than anxiety alone.

Beneficial therapies included L. helveticus R0052 and B. longum R0175 at 10 billion cfu per day for 8 weeks. In a similar study from Canada in this review, there was no evidence that the probiotic formulation was effective in treating low mood; however, this study only used 3 billion units daily of the same probiotics. In studies with probiotics, we often see dose-dependent effects like this.

Other positive studies used L. plantarum 299v at 100 billion cfu twice daily; L. acidophilus, L. casei, and F. bifidum all at 2 billion cfu each daily; and 18 billion cfu of B. bifidum, B. longum, B. lactis, and L. acidophilus. This last combination was used with and without the antidepressant Sertraline. It was found that probiotics improved depression scores.

In another review study, 19 studies were reviewed, covering over 1900 patients. This study also found a benefit with probiotics for major depressive disorder, but not for other clinical disorders. There was also a benefit shown with multistrain probiotics rather than single-strain preparations.[17,18]

One of the proposed mechanisms of probiotics in alleviating depression symptoms is the increased production of tryptophan, which in turn is converted to serotonin. The increase in serotonin that is often reduced in depression helps facilitate better regulation of the patient's symptoms.[19,20]

The latest review article (2022) showed that probiotic rather than prebiotic treatment showed a modest benefit in reducing depression symptoms in major depressive disorder in a period of 4–9 months. Most studies used Lactobacillus or Bifidobacterium.[21]

If you're wondering what probiotic is on the market to save time finding the exact one, Calm Biotic and Probiotic Sticks (Lallemand Health Solutions and Jamieson) are available, with Health Canada approving the latter for the indication of stress, anxiety, and mood balance with level II evidence.

Chapter 6

BACTERIAL VAGINOSIS/ VULVOVAGINAL CANDIDIASIS (YEAST INFECTION)

Bacterial vaginosis (BV) is a rather common condition affecting up to 70% of childbearing women in the US and one of the most common causes of vaginitis symptoms. Simply put, it is an overgrowth of vaginal flora. One type of normal flora that is missing in BV is lactobacilli. Some treatments have focused on replenishing the lactobacilli species to correct or prevent BV. Although some cases can resolve on their own without treatment, antibiotics are normally given to treat them, although recurrence is not uncommon. Some present with no symptoms at all, while others may experience vaginal discharge, odour, and irritation with an altered vaginal pH. Lactobacilli is typically responsible for raising this pH into a less acidic range and preventing the overgrowth of offending flora.

The two main routes of treatment for the prevention of recurrent BV are the oral and vaginal routes. The orally administered route will introduce probiotics vaginally when they pass through the GI system rectally. The vaginal route is preferred since it directly introduces the probiotic vaginally. Lactobacillus doses of 100 billion CFU's for 2 months reduced the recurrence of BV when originally treated with antibiotics. [22]

This would show promise in reducing antibiotic use, which in turn would contribute to reducing antibiotic resistance. As well, BV is a risk factor for acquiring further infections due to an altered immune system pathway.

Further-reaching studies have looked at the effect of probiotics in either treatment or prevention of recurrence of not just BV but also vulvovaginal candidiasis (VVC) commonly known as vaginal yeast infection in the public) and urinary tract infections (UTI's). The key findings are often that although there is certainly an effect with probiotics with or without standard pharmacological treatment in these areas, there is more work to be done on the exact strain or strains and studies that look at long-term effect (over 6 months) are often lacking. In fact, some studies found that the 6-month time frame There is a question about whether probiotics have any effect on recurrence. Regardless of this message, regarding yeast infections, lactobacillus again has proven promise in not only preventing recurrence but also in improving cure rates with conventional medical treatments. Most studies included direct vaginal application of probiotics, although some had oral use. Using probiotics significantly accelerated the return to normal flora within the first month of treatment, but overall, most patients had returned to their normal vaginal flora by the 6-month mark.[23]

A Cochrane review in 2017 on vaginal yeast infections looked at 10 trials with over 1600 patients that lasted from 3 months to 5 years. It found that adding probiotics to standard treatment improved the rate of cure and helped prevent relapse compared to standard treatment alone. Due to the low quality of the evidence, they stopped short of recommending probiotics as add-ons to traditional therapy.[24,25]

A promising new product called Lactin-V has been tested for women who have been treated for a recurrence of bacterial vaginosis. They are given the vaginal preparation containing a human vaginal strain of L. crispatus ctv-05 for 11 weeks. The product showed efficacy at the 3-month check-up time frame. This is actually a "live biotherapeutic product" (LBP) rather than a probiotic.[26,27]

This product represents an interesting change from more standardized products that introduce a specific flora to the body. CTV-05 is a specific strain isolated from the vagina of a healthy woman. It differs from other Lactobacillus strains in that it is a vaginal strain of Lactobacillus. It is resistant to metronidazole, the main treatment for bacterial vaginosis, and may potentially prevent the colonization of many urogenital pathogens. It has also been shown to prevent urinary tract infections. An LBP is a product that is not a vaccine, contains live microorganisms like bacteria, and is applicable to the prevention, treatment, or cure of a disease or condition in humans. It represents the next step in the healthy repopulation of the microbiome and the production of these products for public use.[28]

For the consumer, the more conventional probiotic brands available for BV are Provacare, Ultraflora Women's, and RepHresh Pro B probiotics, which have the strains I've discussed as efficacious for bacterial vaginosis with Health Canada approval for this indication and Level I evidence to back it up. Also, Probaclac BV is Health Canada-approved with level II evidence.

For vaginal candidiasis (yeast infection), the same product recommendation goes with the exception of Probaclac.

One other women's health probiotic of note is for mastitis, an inflammation of the breast tissue that sometimes involves infection and mainly affects breast-feeding women. Materna Opti-Lac Breast Feeding Support has Health Canada approval for this condition with level one evidence. This uses a lactobacillus strain of probiotic that is isolated from breast milk.

Chapter 7

UNVEILING URINARY TRACT INFECTIONS (UTI'S)

In searching for studies on the prevention of UTI's with probiotics, the main problem is the small number of well-designed studies. There has been some work done here, however, that begins to shed light on the role probiotics play in preventing UTI's. There have been various properties proposed that the probiotic should have to give it more success in doing this. They should have good adherence to cells while at the same time preventing the adherence of pathogenic organisms to cells. They should be non-pathogenic themselves and generally safe for the patient to take. They should be able to form clusters as in a normal flora environment and should secrete compounds that prevent the growth of pathogens like hydrogen peroxide and acids.

What has been found is that oral or vaginal administration of different lactobacillus species has shown effectiveness in preventing recurrent urinary tract infections in post-menopausal women, who are often low in lactobacillus in the bladder due to possibly decreased estrogen levels.[29]

A pilot study evaluating the safety and effectiveness of Lactobacillus vaginal suppositories in patients with recurrent urinary tract infections.[30]

Used doses ranging from a million to 100 million CFU's for 4 days to 19 months. Specifically, lactobacillus species that worked best were L. rhamnosus GR-1, L. reuteri, L. crispatis CTV-05, L. rhamnosus GR-1, and L. fermentum B-54. Side effects were typically light.[31,32]

Overall, we are learning more and more that probiotics can play a role in recurrent UTIs, but it isn't as simple as just picking up a bottle of probiotics and hoping for the best.[33]

The reasons for bladder infections are many, and the risk factors for recurrent UTI are not the same between pre- and post-menopausal women. Given this information, it is easier to understand why one species of probiotic might work for one population and then not for another. This is another reason why studies and recommendations need to be specific as to the intended population they will work with. There appears to be an advantage to the vaginal route over the oral route, but there is growing interest in direct instillation into the bladder to more successfully colonize this area. This may prove to be a more challenging route for patients, however. Probiotics overall can offer a relatively safe means of prevention with a low incidence of side effects.

One earlier review in 2006 found that the most encouraging findings were with Lactobacillus rhamnousus GR-1 and L. reuteri RC-14.[34]

Chapter 8

CERVICAL CANCER AWARENESS

Although there appears to be a link between probiotic intake and cancer progression, this information is in its infancy, and what we can say is that there is no firm recommendation to give with respect to an outcome after taking probiotics to prevent cervical cancer. No doubt, this is a field where we will see more work done in the future. If someone tries to convince you that cancer can be treated with probiotics or that the progression of the cancer can be changed with probiotics, you can tell them that we really don't have any proof of that yet, but we are working on it. Nothing would make us happier than to know that probiotics help with cancer risk or progression. We just aren't there yet.

There has been some work on the use of probiotics and their relation to cervical cancer. To start here, there is no recommendation or evidence that tells us to treat cervical cancer with probiotics. I include it here merely as a discussion point, as it may come up to some readers, and I want you to make an informed and correct decision. What is true is that we have evidence that when infected with HPV, the virus that causes cervical cancer, there is a change in the normal flora in the vagina and an increase in adhesion of abnormal flora. Simply speaking, it is believed that this change helps to develop an environment where cervical cancer can develop. There is also work being done that shows the reduction in Lactobacillus species has a detrimental effect on the development of cancer via numerous pathways.[35]

Chapter 9

STRATEGIES FOR EFFECTIVE WEIGHT LOSS

The Centres for Disease Control and Prevention's National Health and Nutrition Examination survey has placed nearly half of the US population over 20 years of age as obese and nearly 80% overweight. This survey was cut short due to COVID, so the numbers are conservative. In Canada, the numbers are slightly lower (just under 70% overweight and obese). The cost involved in handling the medical issues is astronomical. Unfortunately, many recommendations on weight loss via diet plans or gimmicks have either no evidence at all or scarce evidence beyond a 6- to 2-month mark. Also compounding the problem is the stigma involved in weight loss and obesity. Recommendations that suggest someone simply eat better or exercise more are often based on privileged opinions that forget the patient's individual circumstances of income, race, family life, education, and the availability of healthy food. Including this topic in a probiotic book shouldn't mislead the reader into thinking that the obesity epidemic would be reversed by taking a probiotic pill every day. It is interesting, however, to see what effect probiotics have on a patient's weight.

In a well-designed study of 220 patients, lactobacilli and bifidobacteria were found to help reduce weight in 30- to 65-year olds. This study was done by the company that makes the commercial product, which had 50 billion cfu per dose. The percent loss was greater in overweight subjects and those with higher lipid profiles (cholesterol and triglycerides). Maximum weight losses were 2.5%, and measures of BMI, waist circumference, waist-to-height ratio, blood pressure, lipid profile, and inflammatory markers also improved during the study, which had patients maintain their normal lifestyle for 6 months.[36]

In a meta-analysis that reviewed 26 randomized trials and over 1700 people, Results similar to the previous study were found. Body fat loss was noted only when doses of 10 billion units per day were used, and better results were found when multistrain products were used.[37]

Another systematic review done around the same time surveyed the results of 19 trials that included over 1400 patients. The review looked at the effect of probiotics or synbiotics on weight reduction. It was determined that there was no statistically significant change in weight or BMI, but there was a small change in waist circumference. Overall, it recommended more work needs to be done here before we make recommendations for probiotics for weight loss.

A review done in 2021 looked at 27 articles on probiotics and weight loss in human subjects. Although it made recommendations in its conclusion that more studies that find exact recommendations on strains and doses are needed and that studies should zero in on more specific populations with respect to age and sex, overall, the results on probiotics were quite positive.

In this review, species that proved effective for weight loss, BMI reduction, and waist and hip circumference reduction included

L. gasseri SBT2055, L. cuvatus HY7601, and L. plantarum KY1032. Interesting to note is the potential for L. acidophilus to cause weight gain, mainly due to their lack of ability to metabolize fructose and glucose. However, when combined with L. casei and Bifidobacterium, they result in weight loss.[38]

Remember, if you're using probiotics to lose weight, the percent body weight lost even while maintaining a normal diet and activity levels probably won't get you to where you are hoping to, unless that target is 2% or less of your current body weight. Having said that, the studies done thus far in this space are more than interesting in their outcomes, even though they don't give earth-shattering results to the average person.

Health Canada has approved Ultra Flora Control with level I evidence and HMF Metabolic with level II evidence.

Chapter 10

MANAGING CHOLESTEROL LEVELS

It may seem a stretch to suggest that taking a probiotic has any impact on your lipid profile (cholesterol and triglycerides), but considering there are really two main organs that we use in prescription use to lower your total cholesterol, the liver and intestinal tract, it would make sense that exploring this route with probiotics might yield favourable results. What are some ways that probiotics might affect changes in your cholesterol levels?

One proposed mechanism involves the action probiotics have on bile salts, which are used to absorb fats in the intestines from food we eat. Bile salts are normally circulated from the liver, where they are made from cholesterol, to the intestines, where most are typically reabsorbed and returned to the liver for re-secretion. Some probiotics (lactobacillus and bifidobacterial) act on the bile to prevent this reabsorption back into the body, and the bile salts pass through without getting absorbed and are excreted in the feces. This needs to be replaced by making more bile salts in the liver from cholesterol to replenish the supply lost in the cycle. In this way, taking the right probiotic can result in more bile salts being excreted and more cholesterol being used to replace them, thus removing cholesterol from the circulation. It's a pretty interesting proposed mechanism.[39]

While there are other proposed mechanisms as to why probiotics may lower cholesterol levels, it may be more helpful to look at what actual studies have shown us with respect to more useful targets like cardiovascular outcomes. One such review study completed in 2018 looked at 32 studies that, in total, involved almost 2000 subjects. It found that specific strains could significantly lower total cholesterol levels. Although the authors of the study acknowledged the significant lack of cholesterol-lowering ability in the vast majority of probiotics, they did find L. acidophilus, B. lactis, and L. plantarum. Capsule form worked better than drinks or yogurt.[40]

It can be difficult to imagine how probiotics and the intestinal flora would have any effect on cardiovascular disease. We already know that there can be significant differences in bacterial composition between patients with chronic heart failure and control group patients. We have also seen a drop in specific strains and an increase in others in comparison with control groups with respect to chronic heart failure. Much work has yet to be done in this area, so making direct claims isn't possible, but it has become

There is a Health Canada-approved probiotic with the above-mentioned strains with level II evidence for promoting healthy cholesterol levels in adults called Purica Probiotic Cardio.

Chapter 11

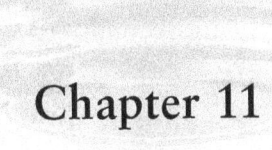

TACKLING ECZEMA

Here is an area where we bring newborns and children into probiotic research and treatment. Although there are several types of eczema, the most common symptoms include itchiness and dry skin, often with scaling patches, but they can also develop into rashes, blisters, and even infections. Sometimes known as atopic dermatitis, where the patient reacts to a trigger, excessive scratching can make this ailment unbearable and can begin as soon as a few weeks after you are born or later on in adulthood. Treatments typically involve antihistamines, steroids, biologics, and other immune-modulating agents, both orally and topically, to help prevent flareups.

Years of research and clinical use of probiotics have been attempted. While today we are still at the "promising evidence shows future potential" phase, as is the case with most probiotic research on various ailments, I have included here some studies that give a mixed conclusion of what we know to date.

A recently completed review of 21 studies looked at the effect of probiotic supplementation both during pregnancy and in the newborn to determine if it reduced the incidence of eczema in the newborn. Compared to the control (placebo) group, the patients treated with various probiotics had a significantly lower chance of eczema and atopic eczema. This effect was even more apparent when multiple strains were used. The effect was even more pronounced when the mother took the probiotics while pregnant rather than just the newborn. The extra symptoms that often go along with dermatitis, including respiratory tract symptoms and allergies, did not seem to be affected in the same manner.[41]

In a study done 7 years earlier, 17 separate studies were looked at that involved a total of 4755 children, divided equally between the probiotic group and the placebo control group. It looked at probiotic supplementation both in pregnancy and after birth and the incidence of several atopic diseases. Overall, it found that eczema development was less in infants of mothers who started probiotics before birth. Conversely, probiotics seemed to have less success in preventing asthma, wheezing, and rhinoconjunctivitis (characterized by nasal congestion, runny nose, sneezing, red eyes, and post-nasal drip, as well as itching of the eyes and nose). Probiotics for prevention of atopic diseases in infants: systematic review and meta-analysis.[42]

Studies that used either Lactobacilli or Bifidobacterium alone had little to no effect, but those that used combination products had a better chance of a positive result. The authors cited a previous meta-analysis that was done a few years earlier and came to similar conclusions, showing a 31% reduction in the incidence of eczema with probiotic use.

The last time that the Cochrane review looked at this topic, their conclusion in 2018 was that the use of probiotics for the treatment of eczema is currently not evidence-based. With this in mind, there really aren't many studies out there testing people with eczema, and the ones available reportedly had results all over the map. It pushed for further study in this space with new probiotics and focused on specific related subgroups in this category, like patients with food allergies, allergic rhinitis, and asthma.

In a 12-week randomized placebo-controlled double-blind study, it was found that Prozema was effective in reducing the amount of topical steroids in children with atopic dermatitis and is Health Canada-approved for Eczema.[43,44]

Chapter 12

EXPLORING THE WORLD OF FERMENTED FOODS AND PREBIOTIC

What if we tried to cultivate the flora of the gut in ways that didn't involve actually taking probiotics? In a world where more and more people want an "all-natural" approach, can we take something that is even more natural than a simple probiotic preparation? It turns out, you can!

While the presence of prebiotics helps to cultivate a person's normal flora, prebiotics are simply a source of food and nutrition for the healthy bacteria in your gut. A better definition is a substrate that is selectively utilized by host microorganisms, conferring a health benefit. Generally, they are carbs that your body won't be able to digest; they travel the length of the digestive system and help to feed your flora as they travel along. Just because something is a dietary fibre doesn't necessarily mean that it is a prebiotic. When we talk of prebiotics, we mainly refer to inulin, fructo-oligosaccharides (FOS), and galacto-oligosaccharides (GOS). Essentially, the bacteria in the gut, in return for this food, are making short-chain fatty acids like butyrate, acetate, and propionate, all good for your health and the health of the cells that line the inside and outside of your gut. As we have discussed, the integrity of this barrier ultimately serves as a gatekeeper to pathways that slowly degrade your health.

Now, regardless of the science on the relationship between probiotics and fibre, we know that increasing the fibre certainly does have proven associations with healthy aging. An estimate from one review study of 25 previous findings was that for every 10 g of fibre in your diet, your risk of colon cancer decreases by about 10%.

What kinds of foods can we ingest that have the fibre that fits this bill? Not all fibres are prebiotics, though. Bananas, apples, pomegranate, nectarines, asparagus, garlic, onions, legumes (red kidney beans, soybeans, chickpeas, and lentils), leeks and shallots, snow peas and green beans, cabbage, whole grains (wheat, barley, and oats), and nuts (pistachios and cashews) are all great sources of prebiotics. Considering that we get about half of the dietary fibre we are supposed to, there is always room for improvement. (cdhf.ca) A dietician is a great source of information on where to start. I filmed a 40-minute, 4-segment video on YouTube at our local grocery store a number of years ago to try and show what's available.[45]

Remember, most recommendations for our health are best taken in moderation, including food recommendations. For example, too much garlic can kill Bifidobacterium, which is a healthy microbe to include in our flora.

Fermented foods are another beneficial intake for those trying to create a more favourable living environment for their normal, healthy flora. They come either in foods or drinks that have been created by microbial growth in a controlled fashion. These include fermented products with probiotics, like some yogurt and some kefir. There are fermented foods with live microbes, like uncooked sauerkraut, kimchi, yogurt, kefir, and most kombuchas. And then there are simple fermented foods without any live microbes, like wine and beer, sourdough bread, tempeh, and chocolate. This may seem confusing when some products have probiotics and some have live microbes. These are not the same. As I mentioned earlier in the book, probiotics are live microorganisms that, when administered in adequate amounts, confer a health benefit on the host. This means, essentially, that probiotics are good bugs or microbes that help us in various aspects of our health. Also, some fermented products don't have enough microbe content to really be called probiotics. The challenge with probiotic foods is that they don't always contain the correct microorganisms or sufficient quantities each time we get a batch to consume. One recommendation of mine is, as always, to check the sugar content of some of these fermented products. While you can't go wrong with consuming most of these fermented products in moderation with a sprinkle of education, the main difference between consuming a probiotic product off the shelf with a stated amount of microbes in it or consuming fermented foods to get your healthy microbe intake is that we don't really have a standardized amount or a high enough amount of probiotics in the fermented food. If you're someone who regularly consumes fermented food with probiotics and prebiotics to cultivate that level of healthy flora, then you may be on your way to a better scenario in the gut. One issue with consuming probiotics willy-nilly is that if you ignore your intake of prebiotics that the organisms need to feed off and survive, they will ultimately take that nourishment from whatever is available in the gut. Potentially, this source could be the mucous layer in your gut. According to the Canadian Digestive Health Foundation, whose association is the Canadian Association of Gastroenterology, This layer in our gut barrier is the primary defence mechanism against harmful compounds that our gut sees every day.

This is a good place to introduce the FODMAP diet. FODMAP is an acronym for fermentable oligosaccharides, disaccharides, monosaccharides, and polyols, and is essentially a group of sugar molecules that most of us consume every day in our carbohydrate intake. Fermentable sugars are digested by bacteria in the intestines. Oligosaccharides can include fructans and galacto-oligosaccharides that aren't absorbed in the small intestine by humans. Disaccharides (two carbohydrate molecules linked together) include the sugar lactose, which needs enzymatic activity from lactase to be absorbed. It isn't uncommon to be deficient in this enzyme and be lactose intolerant. Monosaccharides are sugar molecules found in fruits and vegetables as fructose. When fructose outweighs glucose in a diet, there is a potential for unabsorbed fructose to ferment in the gut, causing IBS symptoms. Polyols are found in low-calorie or sugar-free products and aren't absorbed completely, resulting in adverse GI symptoms.

One of the main groups of patients out there that may be concerned with this information would be those that suffer from IBS, or inflammatory bowel disease. It is thought that up to 50% of people with this affliction Full disclosure here; the evidence on this is not very thorough. The types of carbs in this acronym are merely triggers for those with existing gastrointestinal problems like IBS. Essentially, the sugars included in the FODMAP list aren't well absorbed in the small intestine by some people. This leaves these molecules to travel through the large bowel, where they lead to water being drawn into the colon, and bacteria that naturally occur here begin to ferment the carbohydrates. The by-products of this rapid metabolism include hydrogen and methane. Combining this with the influx of water results in distension of the bowel. Those with IBS don't need much of this distension to happen before it triggers nerve transmission to the network of digestive organs and an overreaction occurs, resulting in characteristic abdominal pain and cramping. Those who consume foods included in the FODMAP diet list are more susceptible to this happening.

My reason for mentioning this here is that some people will try to improve their gut health by consuming some of the FODMAP foods and inevitably feel worse, regardless of their flora makeup. As well, repeated bouts of constipation and diarrhea like those with IBS experience lend themselves to a flora that isn't healthy.

What kinds of food would this include? Unfortunately, it includes a lot of otherwise healthy foods like fruits, vegetables, legumes, milk, and sweeteners. This isn't to say fruits and vegetables cannot be consumed, but they need to be picked from a low-FODMAP diet rather than a high-FODMAP diet. It is beyond the scope of this book to give a complete overview of what to avoid and what to replace it with, but a good dietician can certainly help you make food choices for a more successful trial.

In a small randomized controlled study of about 85 patients, it was found that patients who took a low FODMAP diet with probiotics had no further improvement in symptoms than those who took the same diet with placebo instead. This study used Strep thermophilus, Bifidobacterium lactis and breve, Lactobacillus plantarum, and Acidophilus in CFU strengths in the 100 million ranges.[46]

In a review done the previous year, although results were mixed, it was found that switching to a low FODMAP diet resulted in improvement in symptoms and a change in the microbiome, and when probiotics of various types were given to an IBS patient, symptom improvement was seen.[47]

This probiotic finding was in line with the AEProbio 2023 edition for IBS as well as the Canadian Digestive Health Foundation's recommendations.

PREBIOTICS: FEEDING YOUR GUT MICROBES FOR OPTIMAL HEALTH: INTRODUCTION

If you live in an industrialized society and follow the typical western diet, it is quite possible that some of the residents of your gut microbiome could be considered endangered species. The very changes that have moved us from rural to urban areas, from working on the land to working in office buildings and highly sanitized environments, have not dealt kindly with our resident microbes. This change has resulted in a loss of diversity (both in species and quantity) of bacteria that colonize the gut, but it has also left us deprived of the important benefits provided by the metabolic functions of these microbes. This loss of diversity has wide-ranging implications for our overall health, much of which we are just beginning to understand.

We know they are with us, but where do they live?

Though our digestive tract in its entirety is colonized with microbes, you may be surprised to know that the majority of bacteria that make up our gut microbiome (mostly anaerobes) live in the large intestine, more specifically the colon. Sadly, what often gets lost in the current deluge of marketing and information about gut health is that a diet high in non-digestible carbohydrates, like dietary fibre and prebiotics, provides the very fuel that is essential for these beneficial microbes to thrive.

It should not come as much of a surprise that our traditional western diet does not provide us (or our microbes) with anywhere near enough daily fibre.

The current recommended daily intake of fibre from Health Canada is 25 grams per day for women and 38 grams per day for men. However, most of us are nowhere close to meeting this target. The actual intake of dietary fibre is about 14 grams; the average Canadian daily intake is only about half as much as is recommended.

A lack of dietary fibre has long been linked to a host of problems, much of which are blamed on a phenomenon known as "dysbiosis." Essentially, a diet that is composed of a very low fibre intake can leave our body prone to an imbalance of bacteria in the gut where "bad" bacteria tend to flourish and good bacteria (and the benefits they provide) become compromised.

There is good evidence that dysbiosis is a breeding ground for inflammation, and indeed, dysbiosis has been associated with diseases such as inflammatory bowel disease (IBD), obesity, type 1 and type 2 diabetes, autism, and certain gastrointestinal cancers.

In this chapter, we will further explore the definition, function, benefits, and sources of prebiotics and their impact on our overall health.

PREBIOTICS: A SELECTIVE FOOD FOR GUT BACTERIA

By definition, a prebiotic is "a substrate that is selectively utilized by host microorganisms, conferring a health benefit." In terms of benefit and function, the health benefits of prebiotics are agreed upon to be due to their fermentability by gut microbiota.

This is important because not all forms of fibre can be classified as prebiotic.

Many insoluble fibres cannot be broken down by our digestive system, nor can they be used by our gut bacteria, and thus these types of fibre pass through the gastrointestinal tract unchanged. The majority of the cellulose we ingest, for example, cannot be used as a substrate for gut bacteria; therefore, cellulose is an example of an insoluble fibre that, for the most part, cannot be deemed a prebiotic.

It should be noted that even though non-prebiotic types of fibre may not directly contribute to the gut microbiota or serve as any type of substrate, they still serve a vital purpose in promoting regular bowel movements, enhancing fecal bulk, and blunting the postprandial blood glucose response.

Though this chapter will focus on dietary fibre as a source of prebiotics, it's important to point out that our knowledge about prebiotics is still developing, and there are also non-fibre prebiotic candidates to be aware of, which include lactulose, polyphenols, and polyunsaturated fatty acids.

Among the scientific community, prebiotics are otherwise known as microbiota-accessible carbohydrates (MACs). As stated earlier, MACs are resistant to digestion in the upper gastrointestinal tract; however, in the colon, they serve as food for the bacteria that reside in this part of the gut. Essentially, our gut bacteria are able to feed on these prebiotics and ferment them. The fermentation process gives rise to a variety of molecules that are used both locally in the gut and in other parts of the body. The most notable products of fermentation are short-chain fatty acids. Butyrate, propionate, and acetate account for 90% of the SCFA's produced by the gut microbiota, and over 90% of the SCFA's that are produced in the gut are absorbed and metabolized by either colonocytes (the epithelial cells that line the colon) or the liver, highlighting their ability to act locally but also to cross over from the intestinal lumen to the rest of the body.[48]

WHAT ARE THE BENEFITS?

There is a growing body of evidence supporting the idea that a diet rich in prebiotics has many beneficial effects. Prebiotics and the short-chain fatty acids (SCFA's) that are produced by the fermentation of prebiotics have been shown to have protective effects against colon cancer, reduce both the prevalence and duration of antibiotic-associated diarrhea, and decrease the pH in a specific part of the intestine, thus leading to increased absorption of minerals like calcium and magnesium while reducing the presence of toxic bacterial metabolites and pathogens.

Prebiotics have also demonstrated a beneficial impact on bifidobacteria and lactobacilli, which causes an improvement in fecal bulking, improved bowel movements, immune regulation, and decreased inflammation.

The fermentation of prebiotics and the consequent production of short-chain fatty acids (SCFAs) also lead to a decreased pH in a specific segment of the intestine. This acidic environment promotes increased absorption of essential minerals like calcium and magnesium while reducing the presence of toxic bacterial metabolites and pathogens.

In addition, numerous studies have explored the various benefits of short-chain fatty acids (SCFAs), some of which we will describe briefly here.

At the cellular level, SCFAs have been found to impact various processes, including cell proliferation, differentiation, and gene expression, particularly in relation to energy metabolism, such as lipid metabolism.

We also know that short-chain fatty acids such as butyrate serve as an energy source for both immune cells and the intestinal epithelial cells that line the colon (colonocytes). Butyrate is also important for maintaining intestinal homeostasis through its anti-inflammatory properties and reinforcing gut barrier function.

SCFA's have been shown to have anti-obesity activity by mechanisms that involve appetite suppression and restrained lipogenesis. Their ability to protect against cardiovascular disease by decreasing intestinal cholesterol absorption and possibly even reducing blood pressure has also been observed.

SCFA's may also provide hepatoprotective activity and play an active role in protecting the body from non-viral liver diseases such as alcoholic liver disease (ALD), nonalcoholic fatty liver disease (NAFLD), and drug- or pollutant-induced liver injury. SCFA's have also been shown to have antidiabetic activity by improving insulin sensitivity, improving the balance of glucose in the body, and suppressing the production of glucose by the liver (otherwise known as hepatic gluconeogenesis).

Additional benefits have also been observed in the research, like contributing to longer infant sleep, an ability to increase skeletal muscle mass retention, maintaining healthy bone turnover, and preventing bone loss after menopause.

SCFAs may also have neuroprotective effects. One study conducted on 116 Polish women revealed that those who experienced depression had notably lower levels of acetate and propionate in their stool when compared with that of healthy individuals. Though this is a small study and the authors noted that "no correlations regarding SCFA concentration and fibre intake were found," it does indicate the potential neuroprotective activity of SCFAs.

A recent study on calves also found that enhancing the supply of propionate could alleviate mitochondrial dysfunction, oxidative stress, and apoptosis induced by free fatty acids.

EAT OR BE EATEN.

Essentially, if you do not feed your microbiome, they will not go hungry—at your own expense. Studies have shown that a diet low in prebiotics leads to an increase in mucin-consuming bacteria that essentially begin to eat away at the protective mucosal layer of our intestines. Indeed, those living in western societies tend to have more mucin-ingesting bacteria than those who live in more traditional societies. The implications of this are still being studied; however, there are hypotheses that the consumption of mucin by these bacteria may compromise the permeability of the intestinal wall and thus lead to increased inflammation, as the body interprets this as a possible threat or invasion of the protective layer between the lumen of the intestine and the rest of the body. Some have suggested that this type of scenario could leave the body's immune system predisposed to a state of chronic inflammation, which would have negative effects both on the gut and on the rest of the body.

However, all is certainly not lost. Justin Sonnenberg, a professor of microbiology and immunology at Stanford, has noted that

"DIET is the major tool that we have for manipulating our gut microbiomes in terms of composition and function."

HOW TO FEED YOUR MICROBES:

One way to feed your gut is by increasing your daily intake of fibre-rich fruits and vegetables. In doing this, you will also be increasing your intake of prebiotics.

The most common forms of microbiota-accessible carbohydrates that are able to give rise to short-chain fatty acids exist in the forms of inulin, fructooligosacharides, and resistant starch and can be found in fruits, vegetables, whole grains, nuts, seeds, and legumes. Chicory root, garlic, Jerusalem artichokes, and onions are other examples of foods that are known to contain MACs. It is notable that green bananas are also a source of MACs; however, as they ripen, they unfortunately lose this property.

Though we can acquire prebiotics from various food sources like fruits and vegetables, they are often found in low amounts. Some foods are now prepared with the addition of prebiotics, and there are now prebiotic supplements that may help you reach the recommended dietary intake of 3-5 grams per day (as suggested by the International Scientific Association on Probiotics and Prebiotics).

Unfortunately, you will probably be hard-pressed to find food labels containing the word "prebiotic," but if you look for the actual prebiotic ingredients, you are more likely to find foods that contain them.

Look for these ingredients (Start Low and Go Slow):

- Galactooligossacharides (GOS)
- Fructooligossacharides (FOS)
- Oligofructose
- Chicory Fibre/Root
- Inulin

As pharmacists, we are accustomed to counselling our patients to take a gradual approach to any dietary or lifestyle change. There may be cases in which a patient cannot tolerate certain types of fibre or where a drastic change could result in unwanted side effects such as bothersome gastrointestinal disturbances or a change in medication absorption, and fibre is no exception. It is also important to emphasize that fibre itself can cause constipation if the person is not adequately hydrated. So please do feed your microbes, but if you are just starting out, do so gradually. This will allow your body sufficient time to acclimatize to the introduction of any new foods and hopefully avoid any unwanted or bothersome side effects caused by a drastic change in diet.

In conclusion, prebiotics are an essential component of a healthy diet, promoting the growth of beneficial gut bacteria and leading to numerous health benefits. By feeding our gut microbes with prebiotics and dietary fibre, we can support optimal health for ourselves and future generations.

REFERENCES

How to Manipulate the Microbiota: Prebiotics https://pubmed.ncbi.nlm.nih.gov/27161355/

Prebiotics: Definition, Types, Sources, Mechanisms, and Clinical Applications: https://www.ncbi.nlm.nih.gov/pmc/articles/PMC6463098/#B2-foods-08-00092

Current understanding of dysbiosis in disease in human and animal models: https://www.ncbi.nlm.nih.gov/pmc/articles/PMC4838534/

Expert consensus document: The International Scientific Association for Probiotics and Prebiotics (ISAPP) consensus statement on the definition and scope of prebiotics: https://pubmed.ncbi.nlm.nih.gov/28611480/

Gut-microbiota-targeted diets modulate human immune status. https://pubmed.ncbi.nlm.nih.gov/34256014/

Fermented-food diet increases microbiome diversity and decreases inflammatory proteins, a study finds: https://med.stanford.edu/news/all-news/2021/07/fermented-food-diet-increases-microbiome-diversity-lowers-inflammation

Current understanding of dysbiosis in disease in human and animal models: https://www.ncbi.nlm.nih.gov/pmc/articles/PMC4838534/

How to Manipulate the Microbiota: Prebiotics https://pubmed.ncbi.nlm.nih.gov/27161355/

Prebiotics: Definition, Types, Sources, Mechanisms, and Clinical Applications: https://www.ncbi.nlm.nih.gov/pmc/articles/PMC6463098/#B2-foods-08-00092

Justin Sonnenburg | The Gut Microbiome is a Key Lever on Human Health: https://www.youtube.com/watch?v=yjt26DgVXRc

Should I be eating more fibre? https://www.health.harvard.edu/blog/should-i-be-eating-more-fiber-2019022115927

GOOD GUT ADVICE: EAT MORE FIBRE: https://www.pccmarkets.com/sound-consumer/2016-10/good-gut-advice/

Fibre-Modified Diets: https://www.myrxtx.ca/search

Starving Our Microbial Self: The Deleterious Consequences of a Diet Deficient in Microbiota-Accessible Carbohydrates https://www.ncbi.nlm.nih.gov/pmc/articles/PMC4896489/

Short-Chain Fatty Acids (SCFAs)-Mediated Gut Epithelial and Immune Regulation and Their Relevance for Inflammatory Bowel Diseases: https://www.frontiersin.org/articles/10.3389/fimmu.2019.00277/full

Bélanger, M., Poirier, M., Jbilou, J., & Scarborough, P. (2014). Modelling the impact of compliance with dietary recommendations on cancer and cardiovascular disease mortality in Canada. Public Health, 128(3), 222–230. https://doi.org/10.1016/j.puhe.2013.11.003.

Health Canada (2019) Fibre. Retrieved March 6, 2021, from https://www.canada.ca/en/health-canada/services/nutrients/fibre.html.

Fibre and Whole Grains: https://www.heartandstroke.ca/healthy-living/healthy-eating/fibre-and-whole-grains

Health Benefits and Side Effects of Short-Chain Fatty Acids: https://www.ncbi.nlm.nih.gov/pmc/articles/PMC9498509/

Faecal Short Chain Fatty Acids Profile is Changed in Polish Depressive Women: https://pubmed.ncbi.nlm.nih.gov/30544489/

Propionate alleviates fatty acid-induced mitochondrial dysfunction, oxidative stress, and apoptosis by upregulating PPARG coactivator 1 alpha in hepatocytes. https://pubmed.ncbi.nlm.nih.gov/35181129/

Short-chain fatty acids regulate systemic bone mass and protect from pathological bone loss. https://pubmed.ncbi.nlm.nih.gov/29302038/

Health Benefits and Side Effects of Short-Chain Fatty Acids: https://www.ncbi.nlm.nih.gov/pmc/articles/PMC9498509/#B112-foods-11-02863

POINT COUNTER POINT

Every now and then, there is a post either for or against probiotics with regard to our health. There was a recent exchange that occurred after a Washington Post article written on March 28, 2023, by Anahad O'Connor admitted that probiotics have been found, as I have shown here, to help people with irritable bowel syndrome and inflammatory bowel disease, as well as prevent traveller's diarrhea and some effects of antibiotics. It was also stated correctly that taking probiotics can alter the composition of your microbiome. The article, however, then dives into the threat of dysbiosis and harm. Ironically, on the exact same day, National Geographic published a largely opposing view of probiotics. Both publications agreed that probiotics do have some proven benefits. The difference in the articles was in the stated harms of probiotics and the preferred way to rely on them to nourish the gut.

We are bombarded pretty much daily with information. No other better example than during COVID has we seen that virtually anyone can present a seemingly logical case on almost anything. Oftentimes, when the media gives a message about a study, the full context may be missing. Without having the study in front of them and without knowing how to critically evaluate the study and its power to come to the conclusion it did (something the general public may not know how to do), we are left at the mercy of chance encounters with online messages, newspapers, or broadcast media to do our best in an area that, admittedly, they may not have full knowledge of.

As one of our contributors, Dragana, has said, to say probiotics are healthy for us is like saying medications are healthy for us. Simply taking a probiotic or medication may be completely inappropriate for some. If I told you that I was taking medication from a bottle in the pharmacy and it lowered my cholesterol, you may say, Great, I'm taking something from a bottle in that specific pharmacy, and it should do the same thing. Unfortunately, the bottle you picked was for pinworms and did nothing for your pressure. At this point, you would say that the pharmacy drugs are useless and oversold. This represents one of the most important takeaways in understanding probiotics: a probiotic claim is only as good as the specificity of the strain you are claiming the outcome for. It is also one of the biggest reasons for confusion, not just in the public but also in the medical community, when people are asked for their opinion on the subject. Further complicated is the fact that the blood pressure pill that works for me may not be the one that ends up working for you, or if it does, then the dose may not be the same between each of us. It doesn't mean that the pill doesn't work, but with medicine, we simply accept that there are no guarantees in medicine, and often there is more to a treatment working than one simple medication given to everyone. We are each a system of moving parts that are so plentiful and intertwined that our treatments are often individualized. The unfortunate part is that good therapies are like babies thrown out with the bath water in the interest of discarding false claims or bad science.

To get back to the two opposing probiotic stories, the safety of probiotics should be of prime importance. As I outlined in Healthy Logic (2021), my first priority, either with an OTC selection or a prescription medication, is that the therapy is safe. My second concern is that it works. There is no use in giving a mediation to someone where the risk-benefit ratio rules out giving it in the first place. If you take something and it doesn't work, it shouldn't be dangerous to try that drug. In the journal Gut Microbes, an excellent overview of probiotic safety was given in 2023.[49]

The International Scientific Association for Probiotics and Prebiotics analyzed the quality of the evidence presented in the Washington Post article and declared that there was only one study they were aware of that showed probiotics inhibited microbiome recovery after antibiotic treatment.[50] Furthermore, the actual makeup of our microbiome is much less important than the clinical results (positive or negative) resulting from taking the probiotic.

The International Probiotics Association also responded similarly with the claim that there is no scientific evidence to support the claim that there are a number of health problems due to altered microbial diversity in the gut brought on by taking probiotics. It is also quick to remind us that fermented foods do not mean the same thing as probiotics and that microbes and probiotics are not the same thing.[51]

Overall, the presence of the Post's article online merely served to reinforce a preconceived echo chamber among some health professionals that probiotics are hype. Sadly, they aren't completely wrong, but as health professionals, we can do better by researching a topic as we are trained to. If not, we can at least follow the guidance of professionally recognized groups that state the truth about probiotics: that they do have a place in medicine based on a foundation of science and not opinion.

EFFECT OF PROBIOTICS ON THE METABOLISM OF DRUGS

We have seen how different medications can affect the diversity of our microbiome. Conversely, the microbiome has an effect on the way the body breaks down medications and consequently has the potential to change the effectiveness of medications that we take. Given the fact that dozens of drugs are co-metabolized by the flora found in contact with medications, we can consider the gut microbiome to be a metabolic organ within your body.[52]

One example is statins, the most common family of medications used to lower total and LDL cholesterol. As with other medications, some people have better success than others in lowering cholesterol. It is now suspected that the bile salt levels, which are derived from our microbiome, correlate to a higher level of simvastatin in the blood. Also discovered is that the active form of lovastatin is lower in individuals treated recently with an antibiotic since activation of this drug is carried out by the microbes in the gut. This can help explain the wide range of effects among people on statins based on the possible effect your normal flora has and the fact that everyone's flora isn't the same as someone else's. Also, the effect has limited data for clinical applications but is an important one to have on your radar.

This is just one example of how your normal flora and, consequently, your probiotic and prebiotic intake and your overall diet can have an effect on your therapeutic response to a drug. Other examples of this type of interaction that could lead to a reduction in effect include digoxin for heart function, L-dopa for Parkinson's, ranitidine and omeprazole for reflux and ulcers, loperamide for diarrhea, and indomethacin for pain and inflammation. All have the potential for loss of effect based on the distribution of bacteria in the gut.

Keep in mind right now that, although we are aware in some cases of how specific probiotics can affect the activity of certain medications, we aren't yet at the stage where we can make specific recommendations to correct that. I include it here merely to show the important inclusion we should be showing in the state of the gut in drug response or lack of response. The only common recommendation I give regarding interactions with probiotics is to separate the dose of antibiotic you may be taking from the probiotic so both have the most effect possible.

POSTBIOTICS

The International Scientific Association of Probiotics and Prebiotics has defined a postbiotic as the "preparation of inanimate microorganisms and/or their components that confers a health benefit to the host" If the research into probiotics and prebiotics for our health is a relatively new topic, then postbiotics are even newer and less certain in some ways. But it is not without its research and interesting findings. Postbiotics are essentially what is left in the path of prebiotics and probiotics. It includes cell wall fragments, enzymes, short-chain fatty acids (butyrate), vitamins, amino acids, enzymes, and polysaccharides. Foods that help increase postbiotics in your gut include buttermilk, cottage cheese, oats, seaweed, garlic, fermented pickles, kefir kombucha, tempeh, and fermented sauerkraut.

The debate then becomes: is it the postbiotic material that confers the results we are seeing in studies relating probiotic effects to medical condition improvement, and if that is the case, should we just supplement with postbiotics instead? One of the postbiotics we see is butyrate, which is a key ingredient for gut health and provides the main energy source for your colon cells. These cells get up to 70% of their energy needs from this short-chain fatty acid. As a compounding pharmacist, I have made butyrate enemas for patients prescribed for their gut health.

If you're wondering what you should eat to increase butyrate levels, look back to the prebiotic recommendations I mentioned earlier. Fermentable fibre sources are what you should be looking for. This includes fruit, vegetables, whole grains, and legumes. Many fruits, like apples, apricots, bananas, pears, kiwis, and raspberries, are good choices, as are vegetables like broccoli, carrots, chickpeas, green peas, and potatoes. Foods that are full-fat dairy products are a double-edged sword because of their high saturated fat content and cholesterol, which can have negative cardiovascular effects but do contain butyrate, like butter, cheese, ghee, and milk. The bulletproof coffee fad included butter in your coffee with oil like medium-chain triglyceride oil, but the claims of hunger reduction, weight loss, and mental clarity aren't really backed up by science, and in excess, they were giving people too much saturated fat in some cases.

In another 10 years, there may be enough information out there to write an entire book on postbiotics with the ability to give firm medical recommendations. Many studies on postbiotics and their potential benefits with respect to medical problems focus more on the actual postbiotic ingredient intake and not so much on the existing flora of the patients involved. Based on the infancy of this information, I won't bother giving any studies here, but if you want a recommendation, what I can tell you is that the postbiotic recommendation really doesn't waver much from the "eat a healthy and balanced diet" list, as we've been told for years. One benefit of postbiotics is the ability to take them when probiotics aren't recommended, like in immunocompromised patients, and the stability and expiry issues aren't as much of an issue as probiotics.

PROBIOTIC APPLICATIONS IN ADULT HEALTH

Source: AEProbio https://probioticchart.ca/PBCAdultHealth.html?utm_source=adult_ind&utm_medium=civ&utm_campaign=CDN_CHART

Brand Name	Probiotic Strain	Applications (Level of Recommendation)	Dosage Form	CFU/Dose	No of Doses/Day
BioGaia® Protectis® Baby Drops	L. reuteri DSM 17938	AAD - Antibiotic associated diarrhea - Prevention (I) C - Constipation (I)* CE/AD - Childhood eczema/ Atopic dermatitis (II) CID - Common infectious disease - community acquired (I) Colic - Colic (I)* FAP - Functional abdominal pain (I) IBS - Irritable bowel syndrome (I) ID - Infectious diarrhea (I)* NEC* - Necrotizing Enterocolitis (newborn) *as per hospital protocol, not for self-administration (I) Regurg/ GI Mot - Reduces regurgitation/ Improves gastrointestinal motility (I)*	Drops	100M/5drops	5 drops
BioGaia® Protectis® Chewable tabs	L. reuteri DSM 17938	AAD - Antibiotic associated diarrhea - Prevention (I) C - Constipation (I)* CE/AD - Childhood eczema/ Atopic dermatitis (II) CID - Common infectious disease - community acquired (I) Colic - Colic (I) FAP - Functional abdominal pain (I) IBS - Irritable bowel syndrome (I) ID - Infectious diarrhea (I)* Regurg/ GI Mot - Reduces regurgitation/ Improves gastrointestinal motility (I)	Chewable tablet	100M/tablet	1 tablet

Brand Name	Probiotic Strain	Applications (Level of Recommendation)	Dosage Form	CFU/Dose	No of Doses/Day
BioGaia® Protectis® Drops with Vitamin D	L. reuteri DSM 17938	AAD - Antibiotic associated diarrhea - Prevention **(I)** C - Constipation **(I)** CE/AD - Childhood eczema/ Atopic dermatitis **(II)** CID - Common infectious disease - community acquired **(I)** Colic - Colic **(I)** FAP - Functional abdominal pain **(I)** IBS - Irritable bowel syndrome **(I)** ID - Infectious diarrhea **(I)** Regurg/ GI Mot - Reduces regurgitation/ Improves gastrointestinal motility **(I)**	Drops	100M/5drops	5 drops
BioGaia® Junior Tablets with Vitamin D	L. reuteri DSM 17938	AAD - Antibiotic associated diarrhea - Prevention **(I)** C - Constipation **(I)** CE/AD - Childhood eczema/ Atopic dermatitis **(II)** CID - Common infectious disease - community acquired **(I)** Colic - Colic **(I)** FAP - Functional abdominal pain **(I)** IBS - Irritable bowel syndrome **(I)** ID - Infectious diarrhea **(I)** Regurg/ GI Mot - Reduces regurgitation/ Improves gastrointestinal motility **(I)**	Chewable tablet	100M/tablet	1 tablet
BioGaia® ProDentis™	L. reuteri ATCC PTA 5289 L. reuteri DSM 17938	OH - Oral health (reductions of tonsillitis, laryngitis, and dental caries) **(I)**	Lozenge	200M/lozenge	1 lozenge
CulturedCare® Probiotic Gum with BLIS K12®	Streptococcus salivarius K12	OH - Oral health (reductions of tonsillitis, laryngitis, and dental caries) **(II)**	Lozenge	1B/lozenge	1-5 lozenges

Brand Name	Probiotic Strain	Applications (Level of Recommendation)	Dosage Form	CFU/Dose	No of Doses/Day
Culturelle® Kids Daily Probiotic Chewables	L. rhamnosus GG	AAD - Antibiotic associated diarrhea - Prevention (I) CE/AD - Childhood eczema/ Atopic dermatitis (I) CID - Common infectious disease - community acquired (I) FAP - Functional abdominal pain (I) IBS - Irritable bowel syndrome (I) ID - Infectious diarrhea (I) LH - Liver Health (NASH/NAFLD/MHE; as adjunct to standard therapy; see studies for specific population) (II) NI - Nosocomial infections prevention - hospital acquired (I)	Chewable tablet	5B/tablet	2-4 tablets
Culturelle® Kids Daily Probiotic Packets	L. rhamnosus GG	AAD - Antibiotic associated diarrhea - Prevention (I) CE/AD - Childhood eczema/ Atopic dermatitis (I) CID - Common infectious disease - community acquired (I) FAP - Functional abdominal pain (I) IBS - Irritable bowel syndrome (I) ID - Infectious diarrhea (I) LH - Liver Health (NASH/NAFLD/MHE; as adjunct to standard therapy; see studies for specific population) (II) NI - Nosocomial infections prevention - hospital acquired (I)	Powder	5B/packet	2-4 packets
DanActive® ❄	L. casei sp. paracasei CNCM I-1518	CID - Common infectious disease - community acquired (I) HP - Helicobacter pylori - Adjunct to standard eradication therapy (I) ID - Infectious diarrhea (II)	Ferm. milk 1q.	10B/serving	1-2 servings

Brand Name	Probiotic Strain	Applications (Level of Recommendation)	Dosage Form	CFU/Dose	No of Doses/Day
Ddrops Baby	B. longum CECT7894/KABP042® P. pentosaceus CECT8330/KABP041®	Colic - Colic (I)	Drops	1B/5 drops	5 drops
FlorastorKids®	Saccharomyces boulardii lyo CNCM I-745	AAD - Antibiotic associated diarrhea - Prevention (I) CDAD - Clostridium difficile associated diarrhea - Prevention (III) HP - Helicobacter pylori - Adjunct to standard eradication therapy (I) ID - Infectious diarrhea (I)	Sachet Capsule	5B/sachet 5B/capsule	1-2 sachets 1-2 capsules
Gerber® Baby Cereals	B. lactis BB-12	AAD - Antibiotic associated diarrhea - Prevention (I) CID - Common infectious disease - community acquired (I)	Cereal	1B/serving [serving=5 tbls]	1 serving
Gerber® Toddler Cereals	B. lactis BB-12	AAD - Antibiotic associated diarrhea - Prevention (I) CID - Common infectious disease - community acquired (I)	Cereal	1B/serving [serving=5 tbls]	1 serving
Good Grow® Nutritional Toddler Drink	B. lactis BB-12	AAD - Antibiotic associated diarrhea - Prevention (I) CID - Common infectious disease - community acquired (I)	Powder	1B/200mL serving	1 serving
Good Start Soothe™ Infant Formula	L. reuteri DSM 17938	ID - Infectious diarrhea (I)	Powder	1M/gram	Routine feeding if an alternative to breast milk is required

Brand Name	Probiotic Strain	Applications (Level of Recommendation)	Dosage Form	CFU/Dose	No of Doses/Day
Good Start® Plus 1 Infant Formula	B. lactis BB-12	CID - Common infectious disease - community acquired **(I)**	Powder	1M/gram	Routine feeding if an alternative to breast milk is required
Good Start® Plus 2 Infant Formula *(6 months+)*	B. lactis BB-12	AAD - Antibiotic associated diarrhea - Prevention **(I)** CID - Common infectious disease - community acquired **(I)**	Powder	130M/100mL serving	Routine feeding if an alternative to breast milk is required
HMF Baby Drops	B. longum CECT7894/ KABP042® P. pentosaceus CECT8330/ KABP041®	Colic - Colic **(I)**	Drops	1B/5 drops	5 drops
HMF Fit for School *[50 mg vitamin C, 1000IU vitamin D]*	L. acidophilus CUL-60 L. acidophilus CUL-21 B. animalis subsp. lactis CUL-34 B. bifidum CUL-20	CID - Common infectious disease - community acquired **(I)**	Powder Chewable tablet	12.5B/scoop 12.5B/tablet	1 scoop 1 tablet
MetaKids™ Baby Probiotic	L. rhamnosus GG B. lactis BB-12	CE/AD - Childhood eczema/ Atopic dermatitis **(II)** CID - Common infectious disease - community acquired **(II)**	Drops	1B/6 drops	6 drops
MetaKids™ Probiotic	L. acidophilus NCFM® B. animalis subsp lactis Bi-07®	CID - Common infectious disease - community acquired **(I)**	Chewable tablet	5B/tablet	2 tablets
Nestlé® Nido® Nutritional Toddler Drink	B. lactis BB-12	AAD - Antibiotic associated diarrhea - Prevention **(I)** CID - Common infectious disease - community acquired **(I)**	Powder	1B/200mL serving	1 serving

Brand Name	Probiotic Strain	Applications (Level of Recommendation)	Dosage Form	CFU/Dose	No of Doses/Day
Nutramigen® A+® with LGG® [Branded LGG] *Extensively hydrolyzed casein formula (EHCF)*	L. rhamnosus GG	CMPA - Cow Milk Protein Allergy (including Colic due to CMPA) (I)	Powder	1.35×10^7 CFU per 100 mL serving	EHCF when an alternative to breast milk is required
Orange Naturals Baby Probiotics +D3 Drops (400IU)	L. rhamnosus GG B. lactis BB12	CE/AD - Childhood eczema/ Atopic dermatitis (II) CID - Common infectious disease - community acquired (II)	Drops	2B/5 drops	5 drops
Orange Naturals Probiotics Kids Chewable + Vitamin A,C,D3	L. acidophilus NCFM B. animalis subsp lactis Bi-07	CID - Common infectious disease - community acquired (I)	Chewable tablet	5B/tablet	1 tablet
Probiotic Baby	B. lactis BB-12	CID - Common infectious disease - community acquired (I) Colic - Colic (I)	Drops	1B/6 drops	6 drops
ProZema®	B. lactis BPL1 CECT 8145 B. longum ES1 CECT 7347 L. casei BPL4 CECT 9104	CE/AD - Childhood eczema/ Atopic dermatitis (I)	Stick	1.55B/stick	1 stick
Purica Probiotic Baby Colic	B. longum CECT7894/ KABP042® P. pentosaceus CECT8330/ KABP041®	Colic - Colic (I)	Drops	1B/5 drops	5 drops
Renew Life® FloraBaby	B. breve HA-129 L. rhamnosus HA-111 B. bifidum HA-132 B. infantis HA-116 B. longum HA-135	NEC* - Necrotizing Enterocolitis (newborn) *as per hospital protocol, not for self-administration (II)	Powder	2B/scoop	1-2 scoops
Sisu Probiotic Kid Stiks	L. helveticus R0052 B. infantis R0033 B. bifidum R0071	CID - Common infectious disease - community acquired (I)	Stick	5B/stick	1 stick

PROBIOTIC APPLICATIONS IN VAGINAL HEALTH

Source: AEProbio https://probioticchart.ca/PBCWomensHealth.html?utm_source=women_ind&utm_medium=ciw&utm_campaign=CDN_CHART

Brand Name	Probiotic Strain	Applications (Level of Recommendation)	Dosage Form	CFU/Dose	No. of Doses/Day
Probaclac BV®	L. acidophilus A-212	AAD - Antibiotic associated diarrhea - Prevention **(I)** C - Constipation **(I)** ✱ CE/AD - Childhood eczema/ Atopic dermatitis **(II)** CID - Common infectious disease - community acquired **(I)** Colic - Colic **(I)** ✱	Drops	100M/5drops	5 drops
L. rhamnosus A-119	L. reuteri DSM 17938	FAP - Functional abdominal pain **(I)** IBS - Irritable bowel syndrome **(I)** ID - Infectious diarrhea **(I)** ✱ NEC* - Necrotizing Enterocolitis (newborn) *as per hospital protocol, not for self-administration **(I)** Regurg/ GI Mot - Reduces regurgitation/ Improves gastrointestinal motility **(I)** ✱ AAD - Antibiotic associated diarrhea - Prevention **(I)** C - Constipation **(I)** ✱ CE/AD - Childhood eczema/ Atopic dermatitis **(II)** CID - Common infectious disease - community acquired **(I)** Colic - Colic **(I)** FAP - Functional abdominal pain **(I)** IBS - Irritable bowel syndrome **(I)** ID - Infectious diarrhea **(I)** ✱ Regurg/ GI Mot - Reduces regurgitation/ Improves gastrointestinal motility **(I)**	Chewable tablet	100M/tablet	1 tablet

Brand Name	Probiotic Strain	Applications (Level of Recommendation)	Dosage Form	CFU/Dose	No of Doses/Day
S. thermophilus A-336	BV - Bacterial vaginosis (II) 🌸	Vaginal capsule	8B/capsule	1-2 capsules	
	Provacare®	L. rhamnosus Lcr35	BV - Bacterial vaginosis (I) 🌸		
VC - Vulvovaginal candidiasis (I) 🌸	Vaginal ovule	3.41B/ovule	2 ovules		
	RepHresh™ Pro-B™ Probiotic	L. rhamnosus GR-1			
L. reuteri RC-14	BV - Bacterial vaginosis (I) 🌸				
VC - Vulvovaginal candidiasis (I) 🌸	Oral capsule	0.5B each/capsule		2-4 capsules	
	UltraFlora® Women's 🌸	L. reuteri RC-14			
L. rhamnosus GR-1	BV - Bacterial vaginosis (I) 🌸				
VC - Vulvovaginal candidiasis (I) 🌸	Oral capsule	1B each/capsule	2 capsules		

PROBIOTIC APPLICATIONS IN PEDIATRIC HEALTH

Source: AEProbio https://probioticchart.ca/PBCPediatricHealth.html?utm_source=pediatric_ind&utm_medium=civ&utm_campaign=CDN_CHART

Brand Name	Probiotic Strain	Applications (Level of Recommendation)	Dosage Form	CFU/Dose	No of Doses/Day
BioGaia® Protectis® Baby Drops	L. reuteri DSM 17938	AAD - Antibiotic associated diarrhea - Prevention (I) C - Constipation (I) * CE/AD - Childhood eczema/ Atopic dermatitis (II) CID - Common infectious disease - community acquired (I) Colic - Colic (I) * FAP - Functional abdominal pain (I) IBS - Irritable bowel syndrome (I) ID - Infectious diarrhea (I) * NEC* - Necrotizing Enterocolitis (newborn) *as per hospital protocol, not for self-administration (I) Regurg/ GI Mot - Reduces regurgitation/ Improves gastrointestinal motility (I) * AAD - Antibiotic associated diarrhea - Prevention (I)	Drops	100M/5drops	5 drops
BioGaia® Protectis® Chewable tabs	L. reuteri DSM 17938	C - Constipation (I) * CE/AD - Childhood eczema/ Atopic dermatitis (II) CID - Common infectious disease - community acquired (I) Colic - Colic (I) FAP - Functional abdominal pain (I) IBS - Irritable bowel syndrome (I) ID - Infectious diarrhea (I) * Regurg/ GI Mot - Reduces regurgitation/ Improves gastrointestinal motility (I)	Chewable tablet	100M/tablet	1 tablet

Brand Name	Probiotic Strain	Applications (Level of Recommendation)	Dosage Form	CFU/Dose	No of Doses/Day
BioGaia® Protectis® Drops with Vitamin D	L. reuteri DSM 17938	AAD - Antibiotic associated diarrhea - Prevention (I) C - Constipation (I) 🌸 CE/AD - Childhood eczema/ Atopic dermatitis (II) CID - Common infectious disease - community acquired (I) Colic - Colic (I) 🌸 FAP - Functional abdominal pain (I) IBS - Irritable bowel syndrome (I) 🌸 ID - Infectious diarrhea (I) 🌸 Regurg/GI Mot - Reduces regurgitation/ Improves gastrointestinal motility (I) 🌸	Drops	100M/5drops	5 drops
BioGaia® Junior Tablets with Vitamin D	L. reuteri DSM 17938	AAD - Antibiotic associated diarrhea - Prevention (I) C - Constipation (I) 🌸 CE/AD - Childhood eczema/ Atopic dermatitis (II) CID - Common infectious disease - community acquired (I) Colic - Colic (I) FAP - Functional abdominal pain (I) IBS - Irritable bowel syndrome (I) ID - Infectious diarrhea (I) 🌸 Regurg/GI Mot - Reduces regurgitation/ Improves gastrointestinal motility (I)	Chewable tablet	100M/tablet	1 tablet
BioGaia® ProDentis™	L. reuteri ATCC PTA 5289 L. reuteri DSM 17938	OH - Oral health (reductions of tonsillitis, laryngitis, and dental caries) (I) 🌸	Lozenge	200M/lozenge	1 lozenge
CulturedCare® Probiotic Gum with BLIS K12®	Streptococcus salivarius K12	OH - Oral health (reductions of tonsillitis, laryngitis, and dental caries) (II) 🌸	Lozenge	1B/lozenge	1-5 lozenges

CHAPTER 12: EXPLORING THE WORLD OF FERMENTED FOODS AND PREBIOTIC | 107

Brand Name	Probiotic Strain	Applications (Level of Recommendation)	Dosage Form	CFU/Dose	No of Doses/Day
Culturelle® Kids Daily Probiotic Chewables	L. rhamnosus GG	AAD - Antibiotic associated diarrhea - Prevention **(I)** CE/AD - Childhood eczema/ Atopic dermatitis **(I)** CID - Common infectious disease - community acquired **(I)** FAP - Functional abdominal pain **(I)** IBS - Irritable bowel syndrome **(I)** ID - Infectious diarrhea **(I)** LH - Liver Health (NASH/NAFLD/MHE; as adjunct to standard therapy; see studies for specific population) **(II)** NI - Nosocomial infections prevention - hospital acquired **(I)**	Chewable tablet	5B/tablet	2-4 tablets
Culturelle® Kids Daily Probiotic Packets	L. rhamnosus GG	AAD - Antibiotic associated diarrhea - Prevention **(I)** CE/AD - Childhood eczema/ Atopic dermatitis **(I)** CID - Common infectious disease - community acquired **(I)** FAP - Functional abdominal pain **(I)** IBS - Irritable bowel syndrome **(I)** ID - Infectious diarrhea **(I)** LH - Liver Health (NASH/NAFLD/MHE; as adjunct to standard therapy; see studies for specific population) **(II)** NI - Nosocomial infections prevention - hospital acquired **(I)**	Powder	5B/packet	2-4 packets
DanActive® ♣ ✽	L. casei sp. paracasei CNCM I-1518	CID - Common infectious disease - community acquired **(I)** HP - Helicobacter pylori - Adjunct to standard eradication therapy **(I)** ID - Infectious diarrhea **(II)**	Ferm. milk lq.	10B/serving	1-2 servings

Brand Name	Probiotic Strain	Applications (Level of Recommendation)	Dosage Form	CFU/Dose	No of Doses/Day
Ddrops Baby	B. longum CECT7894/KABP042® P. pentosaceus CECT8330/KABP041®	Colic - Colic (I)	Drops	1B/5 drops	5 drops
FlorastorKids®	Saccharomyces boulardii lyo CNCM I-745	AAD - Antibiotic associated diarrhea - Prevention (I) CDAD - Clostridium difficile associated diarrhea - Prevention (III) HP - Helicobacter pylori - Adjunct to standard eradication therapy (I) ID - Infectious diarrhea (I) AAD - Antibiotic associated diarrhea - Prevention (I)	Capsule Sachet	5B/capsule 5B/sachet	1-2 capsules 1-2 sachets
Gerber® Baby Cereals	B. lactis BB-12	CID - Common infectious disease - community acquired (I) AAD - Antibiotic associated diarrhea - Prevention (I)	Cereal	1B/serving [serving=5 tbls]	1 serving
Gerber® Toddler Cereals	B. lactis BB-12	CID - Common infectious disease - community acquired (I) AAD - Antibiotic associated diarrhea - Prevention (I)	Cereal	1B/serving [serving=5 tbls]	1 serving
Good Grow® Nutritional Toddler Drink	B. lactis BB-12	CID - Common infectious disease - community acquired (I)	Powder	1B/200mL serving	1 serving
Good Start Soothe™ Infant Formula	L. reuteri DSM 17938	ID - Infectious diarrhea (I)	Powder	1M/gram	Routine feeding if an alternative to breast milk is required
Good Start® Plus 1 Infant Formula	B. lactis BB-12	CID - Common infectious disease - community acquired (I)	Powder	1M/gram	Routine feeding if an alternative to breast milk is required

Brand Name	Probiotic Strain	Applications (Level of Recommendation)	Dosage Form	CFU/Dose	No of Doses/Day
Good Start® Plus 2 Infant Formula (6 months+)	B. lactis BB-12	AAD - Antibiotic associated diarrhea - Prevention **(I)** CID - Common infectious disease - community acquired **(I)**	Powder	130M/100mL serving	Routine feeding if an alternative to breast milk is required
HMF Baby Drops	B. longum CECT7894/ KABP042® P. pentosaceus CECT8330/ KABP041®	Colic - Colic **(I)**	Drops	1B/5 drops	5 drops
HMF Fit for School *[50 mg vitamin C, 1000IU vitamin D]*	L. acidophilus CUL-60 L. acidophilus CUL-21 B. animalis subsp. lactis CUL-34 B. bifidum CUL-20	CID - Common infectious disease - community acquired **(I)**	Powder Chewable tablet	12.5B/scoop 12.5B/tablet	1 scoop 1 tablet
MetaKids™ Baby Probiotic	L. rhamnosus GG B. lactis BB-12	CE/AD - Childhood eczema/ Atopic dermatitis (II) CID - Common infectious disease - community acquired (II)	Drops	1B/6 drops	6 drops
MetaKids™ Probiotic	L. acidophilus NCFM® B. animalis subsp lactis Bi-07®	CID - Common infectious disease - community acquired **(I)** AAD - Antibiotic associated diarrhea - Prevention **(I)**	Chewable tablet	5B/tablet	2 tablets
Nestlé® Nido® Nutritional Toddler Drink	B. lactis BB-12	CID - Common infectious disease - community acquired **(I)**	Powder	1B/200mL serving	1 serving
Nutramigen® A+® with LGG® *Extensively hydrolyzed casein formula (EHCF)*	L. rhamnosus GG [Branded LGG]	CMPA - Cow Milk Protein Allergy (including Colic due to CMPA) **(I)**	Powder	1.35 × 10⁸ CFU per 100 mL serving	EHCF when an alternative to breast milk is required
Orange Naturals Baby Probiotics +D3 Drops (400IU)®	L.rhamnosus GG B.lactis BB12	CE/AD - Childhood eczema/ Atopic dermatitis (II) CID - Common infectious disease - community acquired (II)	Drops	2B/5 drops	5 drops
Orange Naturals Probiotics Kids Chewable + Vitamin A,C,D3®	L. acidophilus NCFM B. animalis subsp. lactis Bi-07	CID - Common infectious disease - community acquired **(I)**	Chewable tablet	5B/tablet	1 tablet

Brand Name	Probiotic Strain	Applications (Level of Recommendation)	Dosage Form	CFU/Dose	No of Doses/Day
Probiotic Baby	B. lactis BB-12	CID - Common infectious disease - community acquired (I) Colic - Colic (I)	Drops	1B/6 drops	6 drops
ProZema® 🍁	B. lactis BPL1 CECT 8145 B. longum ES1 CECT 7347 L. casei BPL4 CECT 9104 B. longum CECT7894/	CE/AD - Childhood eczema/ Atopic dermatitis (I) 🍁	Stick	1.55B/stick	1 stick
Purica Probiotic Baby Colic 🍁	KABP042® P. pentosaceus CECT8330/ KABP041® B. breve HA-129	Colic - Colic (I) 🍁	Drops	1B/5 drops	5 drops
Renew Life® FloraBaby	L. rhamnosus HA-111 B. bifidum HA-132 B. infantis HA-116 B. longum HA-135 L. helveticus R0052	NEC* - Necrotizing Enterocolitis (newborn) *as per hospital protocol, not for self-administration (II)	Powder	2B/scoop	1-2 scoops
Sisu Probiotic Kid Stiks 🍁	B. infantis R0033 B. bifidum R0071	CID - Common infectious disease - community acquired (I)	Stick	5B/stick	1 stick

Disclaimer: The information is from http://www.aeprobio.com and charts on this website are updated on an annual basis.
*The presence of a maple leaf signifies that it has received approval from Health Canada for the specified condition.

CHAPTER 12: EXPLORING THE WORLD OF FERMENTED FOODS AND PREBIOTIC | 111

To this point, I have tried to give an overview of what is proven and what isn't when it comes to probiotics, prebiotics, postbiotics, and anything else you can introduce into your gut to elicit a positive response for a variety of medical issues. The hope is that this will lead you down a path of healthier outcomes overall and healthier aging. There is no shortage of hype on social media today, but the scientific method has consistently proven to be the best route to take in growing our information. In today's environment, there is a lot of money to be made by those who recognize the acceptance of a large percentage of the general public for a quick fix that medicine has overlooked or not recognized as being effective. As someone who works within the front lines of medicine, I can assure you that no one is withholding any therapy that we know to be safely effective. Executives at drug companies have families too and also want the best for them. Having said that, as a pharmacist, I also fully acknowledge the past wrongdoings of Big Pharma that have left the entire medical community to defend what we do. There is a noticeable separation your doctor and pharmacist would like to observe between making recommendations that are unsafe, expensive, not proven, or outright quackery and those that are not.

This is not to say that everything we recommend to you is off-label, but it must be safe. Off-label prescribing amounts to over 10% of all prescribing in Canada, and over 70% of all pediatric prescribing is off-label, meaning there is no approved use for a product by the company that makes it, either at any age or at a specific age. Some medications make it to national guidelines for their use without actually being approved for their use. It's just standard practice because it works. Some products were initially brought to market for one medical issue and found a niche in another. Some drugs simply weren't tested in clinical trials in the age group or sex they are now comfortably used in. And sometimes there is simply no option other than an off-label drug.

Attempts at off-label use often fall flat, as we have seen during COVID with drugs like hydroxychloroquine or ivermectin. For whatever reason, the administration of medicine can have grey areas, but we should never use that as the sole reason we are selling a product. Making money can be nice, but taking money from people when there is no evidence at all that something works is just wrong. And although anecdotal evidence carries the least weight, most medical professionals often rely on this type of evidence from time to time to refine their prescribing habits or recommendations to the public.

This brings us to the recommendation of probiotics for various health issues. While it is true that some of these recommendations have overspilled in recent years into the realm of unproven money grabs with the hope that a physiologic story and a logical outcome will make sense and work, we now have better evidence that, when taken correctly, a specific probiotic can help you. To have specific outcomes, medicine should be specific, and specific recommendations are needed to give back the credibility that probiotics offer. As we have seen in this book, the world of probiotic recommendations needs very specific recommendations, not only for dosing but for the exact strain that works, not just one that sounds like it or something labelled "probiotics.".

To start with, taking care of your gut is much easier when you don't give it an offensive or damaging agent. This is not to say that something like one drink of alcohol will have long-term consequences for your gut lining, but regular use may. Medications that are taken for pain and inflammation can have a damaging effect on the gut but are sometimes necessary. Medications that cause constipation, like iron, narcotics, some antidepressants, calcium supplements or antacids that contain calcium or aluminium, some blood pressure medications, and some diuretics, can also cause constipation, which has negative effects on bowel health. Check with your pharmacist if you suspect your medications might be the cause of your constipation. Keeping a well-balanced diet with sufficient water and regular exercise may help keep you more regular. Often, extra water intake has little bearing on constipation, but scarce water intake won't help. Antibiotics, while necessary at times, can also adversely affect the bowel by changing the microbiotic makeup in the gut, especially when probiotics are not taken to maintain that. Smoking, heavy metal exposure, and environmental chemicals also contribute negatively to gut health. So, without even supplementing with probiotics, you can positively work on your gut flora by being mindful of all these products. As always, stress is your enemy, and it's no different when it comes to the gut lining.

Another way we discussed without direct supplementation is to feed bacteria already present with prebiotics. This is the food that probiotics live off of. Some of these products are sources of dietary fibre, like chicory root. The majority of chicory root fibre comes from inulin, a prebiotic fibre that helps reduce constipation. Dandelion greens, Jerusalem artichoke, garlic, onions, leeks, asparagus, bananas, barley, oats, cocoa, and flaxseeds are all great sources of prebiotics. Wheat bran is also popular, as is seaweed. As always, try to seek out fermented foods to help with this, like kombucha, miso, yogurt (sugarless), tempeh, kefir, kimchi, sauerkraut, apple cider vinegar, and pickles. Also, remember that even though yogurt has bacteria in it, it isn't necessarily probiotic.

I am often asked about the safety of probiotics for various populations. Based on the history of the use of probiotics, not only as a supplement but also in the use of probiotics in foods over the years, we know that probiotics are quite unlikely to cause harm to those who are using them. It is also negligible how many probiotics have caused opportunistic infections. There doesn't seem to be one case of sepsis in newborns (including premature ones) who have been given probiotics. Probiotics are included in various baby formulas without any infections being noted. For regular adult users of probiotics, side effects are normally quite mild. These are often limited to gastrointestinal symptoms such as gas. In those who are severely ill or immunocompromised, there have been reports of severe illness, and the use of probiotics in these patients should be used with caution and perhaps lean towards prebiotics instead. With regards to pregnancy, studies have shown that probiotics are safe for use during pregnancy, and the side effect profile in this population is also minimal. Are probiotics safe for use during pregnancy and lactation?[53]

Finally, when making actual choices on what probiotic to supplement with, if you choose to do so, remember to stick with the evidence given in each chapter for the various medical issues. Close attention should be given to the exact strain referenced in the chapters. For the best summary of a multitude of indications, refer to aeprobio.com; it's the best reference out there for evidence-based guidelines. If you approach your pharmacist about these products, some specialized companies are out there beyond the ordinary shelf of vitamin and supplement companies. Be sure to purchase a product with a recognized NPN or DIN number to show that it at least has the eyes of your country's drug-regulating body on it. And as always, don't start any long-term (over 7 days) supplement or medication without consulting your doctor or pharmacist. The recommendations I have laid out in this book are hopefully easy for you to follow, not just in prebiotic foods to consume to help feed your microbiome but also with very specific products for various medical conditions. With a small amount of homework, you can be healthier by looking after your gut!

Gut Health Journal

FOOD AND BEVERAGE INTAKE:

Record everything you eat and drink throughout the day. Include details such as portion sizes, meal times, and ingredients. Be specific about the types of foods and beverages consumed.

Note any digestive symptoms or discomfort after meals, such as bloating, gas, diarrhea, or constipation. This information can help you identify potential trigger foods or patterns of gut distress.

PHYSICAL ACTIVITY AND EXERCISE:

Document your daily physical activity and exercise routine. Include details like the type of exercise, duration, and intensity.

Pay attention to how exercise makes you feel in terms of digestion. Note if you experience improved digestion, reduced bloating, or changes in appetite after physical activity.

Emotional Well-Being and Stress:

Keep a record of your daily stress levels and emotional state. Stress can have a significant impact on gut health, so it's essential to monitor and manage it.

Reflect on any stress-reduction techniques you incorporate into your day, such as meditation, deep breathing exercises, or yoga. Note how these practices affect your overall well-being and digestive comfort.

Dragana Skokovic-Sunjic
RPh BScPhm NCMP

Hamilton Family Health Team
Alliance for Education on Probiotics
Hamilton, Ontario
dsunjic@BHSoftInc.com
1-905-966-2803

Dragana Skokovic-Sunjic is a Clinical Pharmacist and NAMS credentialed Menopause Practitioner NCMP, practicing in a primary care setting with Hamilton Family Health Team. In addition to her collaborative clinical practice, she is a leader in knowledge mobilization for probiotics in Canada and the United States.

Translating scientific research in this field, she has authored *'Clinical Guide to Probiotic Supplements Available in Canada'* and *'Clinical Guide to Probiotic Products Available in the US'* since 2008. This practical clinical tool is peer-reviewed and updated annually to reflect the latest evidence and includes available probiotic products in the Canadian and US markets. Dragana's project has been presented, published and recognized internationally, receiving numerous awards and recognition.

The Canadian version of the Clinical Guide to Probiotics can be found at www.ProbioticChart.ca and the US version at www.USProbioticGuide.com

Dragana's efforts to promote evidence-based education in this field resulted in establishing the Alliance for Education on Probiotics or AEProbio™ in 2015. AEProbio supports publishing the Clinical Guides to Probiotic Products and coordinates the preparation and delivery of various educational pieces designed for healthcare professionals and consumers.

The summary of the educational offerings can be found at www.AEProbio.com

Dragana's objective is to enable clinicians and patients to recognize if and when probiotic therapy is necessary and what particular strain(s) would be the most appropriate for the desired outcome.

Dragana has collaborated and coauthored books and publications in the area of public health, probiotics, women's health and more. She is a guest lecturer at the Pharmacy School, University of Waterloo in Ontario, McMaster University Medical Residents, Hamilton, Ontario.

Dragana's probiotic project has been featured in the Washington Post, New York Times, Forbes, National Geographic, CBC, and more.

Lindsay Dixon
RPh BScPhm

Lindsay Dixon is a registered Pharmacist from Victoria, British Columbia, where she currently works with Heart Pharmacy Group. Lindsay has practiced pharmacy for over 10 years, the majority of which has been in the area of Community Pharmacy Management.

In March of 2020, Lindsay founded Friendly Pharmacy 5 - a multimedia platform where Lindsay harnesses the power of video to communicate evidence-based science to the public and provide viewers with credible, easy to understand health information. This work has led to countless media engagements, and collaborations with scientists and healthcare professionals both nationally and internationally.

In 2021, Lindsay was awarded the Ben Gant Innovative practice award from the BC Pharmacy Association for her multimedia work throughout the pandemic and in 2022 she was recognized by Pharmacy Practice & Business Magazine with the Raise Your Voice Award, again for her multimedia work. Lindsay's videos and blog posts are also featured regularly on the Canadian Healthcare Network.

Lindsay is most passionate about equipping the public to make informed choices about their own health by providing them with credible, science-based resources and education.

ABOUT THE AUTHOR

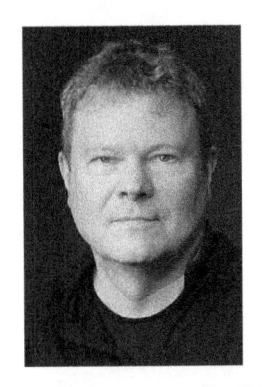

Graham graduated with a BSc in chemistry from St Francis Xavier University in Antigonish, Nova Scotia in1989 before entering Pharmacy at Dalhousie University in Halifax. His chemistry background has grown into a strong involvement in compounding in his Pharmacy. Graham graduated from Dalhousie College of Pharmacy in Halifax, NS in 1993. Immediately after graduation he returned to his roots on Cape Breton Island and went to work in Baddeck at Stone's Drug Store. In 2001, Graham purchased the pharmacy and since then there have been many changes made over the years. Today, there is a compounding lab, a nursing home packaging area, and a private consultation room. As his practice has evolved, Graham has drawn definitive – and sometimes controversial – lines around what he can ethically sell in his store. He opted to stop selling sugary beverages in 2014 and removed all homeopathic products from his shelves in 2018. He has also become involved in clinical studies to forward the scientific community's understanding of pain compounding salves. Graham will always be a pharmacist first, but he is also a healthcare professional who unapologetically aims to guide both his customers and his readers to make better decisions about medication, diet, and healthy living.

Endnotes

1. Joint FAO/WHO Expert Consultation on Evaluation of Health and Nutritional Properties of Probiotics in Food, including Powder Milk with Live Lactic Acid Bacteria, 1-4 October 2001
2. Hill, C., Guarner, F., Reid, G., et al., The International Scientific Association for Probiotics and Prebiotics consensus statement on the scope and appropriate use of the term probiotic. Nat Rev Gastroenterol Hepatol 11, 506–514 (2014) https://doi.org/10.1038/nrgastro.2014.66
3. Skokovic-Sunjic, D. Clinical Guide to Probiotic Products) Available in the United States: 8th Edition, 2023, February 2023, AEProbio (BH Soft Inc., ISBN: 978-1-7775181-5-8).
4. I, Microbiome: A Secret to a Healthy and Balanced Human Body, V. Jakovljevic et al., 2023). Lets Author
5. https://www.sciencedaily.com/releases/2021/02/210203090458.htm
6. Int J Mol Sci. 2017 Dec 7;18(12):2645
7. https://www.cochranelibrary.com/cdsr/doi/10.1002/14651858.CD006895.pub4/full
8. https://www.cochranelibrary.com/cdsr/doi/10.1002/14651858.CD009066.pub2/full
9. Garaiova I, Muchová J, Nagyová Z, Wang D, Li JV, Országhová Z, Michael DR, Plummer SF, Ďuračková Z. Probiotics and vitamin C for the prevention of respiratory tract infections in children attending preschool: a randomized controlled pilot study Eur J Clin Nutr. 2015 Mar;69(3):373-9. doi: 10.1038/ejcn.2014.174. Epub 2014 Sep 10. PMID: 25205320; PMCID: PMC4351422.
10. https://journals.lww.com/md-journal/Fulltext/2019/09130/A_meta_analysis_of_the_effects_of_probiotics_and.1.aspx
11. https://www.cochrane.org/CD004827/IBD_probiotics-prevention-antibiotic-associated-diarrhea-children
12. https://www.cochrane.org/CD006095/IBD_use-probiotics-prevent-clostridium-difficile-diarrhea-associated-antibiotic-use
13. Harper A., Naghibi MM, and Garcha D., The Role of Bacteria, Probiotics, and Diet in Irritable Bowel Syndrome. Foods. 2018 Jan 26;7(2):13. doi: 10.3390/foods7020013. PMID: 29373532; PMCID: PMC5848117.
14. Gut Microbes. 2016; 7(5): 365–383.
15. Published online on July 29, 2016. doi: 10.1080/19490976.2016.1218585

16 Front. Neurol., 22 May 2020, Sec. NeuropharmacologyVolume 11: 2020 | https://doi.org/10.3389/fneur.2020.00421

17 Kah Kheng Goh, Yen-Wenn Liu, Po-Hsiu Kuo, Yu-Chu Ella Chung, Mong-Liang Lu, Chun-Hsin Chen,

18 Effect of probiotics on depressive symptoms: A meta-analysis of human studies, Psychiatry Research,Volume 282, 2019

19 Ann Gen Psychiatry 16, 14 (2017). https://doi.org/10.1186/s12991-017-0138-2

20 Wallace, C.J.K., and Milev, R. The effects of probiotics on depressive symptoms in humans: a systematic review.

21 Alli SR, Gorbovskaya I, Liu JCW, Kolla NJ, Brown L, Müller DJ) The Gut Microbiome in Depression and the Potential Benefits of Prebiotics, Probiotics, and Synbiotics: A Systematic Review of Clinical Trials and Observational Studies International Journal of Molecular Sciences, 2022, 23(9):4494. https://doi.org/10.3390/ijms23094494

22 Webb, Lauren, DMSc, PA-C. Probiotics for preventing recurrent bacterial vaginosis JAAPA 34(2):p 19-22, February 2021. | DOI: 10.1097/01.JAA.0000731484.81301.58

23 Jeng, H., Yan, T., and Chen, J. Treating vaginitis with probiotics in nonpregnant females: A systematic review and meta-analysis." Experimental and Therapeutic Medicine 20.4 (2020): 3749–3765

24 Cochrane Database of Systematic Reviews 2017, Issue 11. Art. No.: CD010496. DOI: 10.1002/14651858.CD010496.pub2).

25 Xie H, Feng D, Wei D, Mei L, Chen H, Wang X, and Fang F. Probiotics for vulvovaginal candidiasis in non-pregnant women.

26 VOLUME 3, ISSUE 6, E435-E442, JUNE 2022) Sustained effect of LACTIN-V (Lactobacillus crispatus CTV-05) on genital immunology following standard bacterial vaginosis treatment: results from a randomized, placebo-controlled trial, Eric Armstrong, BSc, et al. Open Access Published:April 21, 2022 DOI:https://doi.org/10.1016/S2666-5247(22)00043-X)

27 Cohen,C.R. M.D. et al. Randomized Trial of Lactin-V to Prevent Recurrence of Bacterial Vaginosis, N EnglMed2020; 382:1906–1915 DOI: 10.1056/NEJMoa1915254

28 Lagenaur LA, Hemmerling A, Chiu C, Miller S, Lee PP, Cohen CR, and Parks TP Connecting the Dots: Translating the Vaginal Microbiome Into a Drug J Infect Dis. 2021 Jun 16;223(12 Suppl 2):S296-S306. doi: 10.1093/infdis/jiaa676. PMID: 33330916; PMCID: PMC8502429.

29 Shinya Uehara, Koichi Monden, Koji Nomoto, Yuko Seno, Reiko Kariyama, Hiromi Kumon

30 International Journal of Antimicrobial Agents, Volume 28, Supplement 1, 2006, Pages 30-34
31 Turk J Urol. 2018 Sep;44(5):377–383. doi: 10.5152/tud.2018.48742. Epub 2018 Sep 1. PMID: 30487041; PMCID: PMC6134985.
32 Akgül T., Karakan T. The role of probiotics in women with recurrent urinary tract infections.
33 (Abdullatif V A, Sur R L, Eshaghian E, et al. (October 17, 2021): Efficacy of Probiotics as Prophylaxis for Urinary Tract Infections in Premenopausal Women: A Systematic Review and Meta-Analysis. Cureus 13(10): e18843 (doi:10.7759/cureus.18843)
34 Falagas, M.E., Betsi, G.I., Tokas, T., et al., Probiotics for Prevention of Recurrent Urinary Tract Infections in Women, Drugs 66, 1253–1261 (2006). https://doi.org/10.2165/00003495-200666090-00007)
35 Front. Cell. Infect. Microbiol., 28 July 2022Sec. Microbiome in Health and DiseaseVolume 12: 2022 | https://doi.org/10.3389/fcimb.2022.963868
36 Michael DR, Jack AA, Masetti G, Davies TS, Loxley KE, Kerry-Smith J, Plummer JF, Marchesi JR, Mullish BH, McDonald JAK, Hughes TR, Wang D, Garaiova I, Paduchová Z, Muchová J, Good MA, Plummer SF) A randomized controlled study shows supplementation of overweight and obese adults with lactobacilli and bifidobacteria reduces bodyweight and improves well-being. Sci Rep. 2020 Mar 6;10(1):4183. doi: 10.1038/s41598-020-60991-7. PMID: 32144319; PMCID: PMC7060206.
37 Pontes KSDS, Guedes MR, Cunha MRD, Mattos SS, Barreto Silva MI, Neves MF, Marques BCAA, Klein MRST) Effects of probiotics on body adiposity and cardiovascular risk markers in individuals with overweight and obesity: A systematic review and meta-analysis of randomized controlled trials Clin Nutr. 2021 Aug;40(8):4915-4931. doi: 10.1016/j.clnu.2021.06.023. Epub 2021 Jul 3. PMID: 34358838.
38 Álvarez-Arraño, V.; Martín-Peláez, S. Effects of Probiotics and Synbiotics on Weight Loss in Subjects with Overweight or Obesity: A Systematic Review. Nutrients 2021, 13, 3627 https://doi.org/10.3390/ nu13103627
39 Reis SA, Conceição LL, Rosa DD, Siqueira NP, Peluzio MCG) Mechanisms responsible for the hypocholesterolaemic effect of regular consumption of probiotics Nutr Res Rev. 2017 Jun;30(1):36-49. doi: 10.1017/S0954422416000226. Epub 2016 Dec 20. PMID: 27995830.
40 Wang L, Guo MJ, Gao Q, Yang JF, Yang L, Pang XL, and Jiang XJ. The effects of probiotics on total cholesterol: A meta-analysis of randomized controlled trials Medicine (Baltimore). 2018 Feb;97(5):e9679. doi: 10.1097/MD.0000000000009679. PMID: 29384846; PMCID: PMC5805418.

41 Shuya Sun, Guizhen Chang, and Litao Zhang (2022), The prevention effect of probiotics against eczema in children: an update, systematic review, and meta-analysis, Journal of Dermatological Treatment, 33:4, 1844–1854. DOI: 10.1080/09546634.2021.1925077

42 G. Zuccotti, F. Meneghin, A. Aceti, G. Barone, M. L. Callegari, A. Di Mauro, M. P. Fantini, D. Gori, F. Indrio, L. Maggio, L. Morelli, and L. Corvaglia, on behalf of the Italian Society of Neonatology First published: July 21, 2015 https://doi.org/10.1111/all.12700

43 Navarro-López V, Ramírez-Boscá A, Ramón-Vidal D, Ruzafa-Costas B, Genovés-Martínez S, Chenoll-Cuadros E, Carrión-Gutiérrez M, Horga de la Parte J, Prieto-Merino D, Codoñer-Cortés FM. Effect of Oral Administration of a Mixture of Probiotic Strains on the SCORAD Index and Use of Topical Steroids in Young Patients With Moderate Atopic Dermatitis: A Randomized Clinical Trial JAMA Dermatol. 2018 Jan 1;154(1):37-43. doi: 10.1001/jamadermatol.2017.3647. PMID: 29117309; PMCID: PMC5833582.

44 Tan-Lim CSC, Esteban-Ipac NAR, Recto MST, Castor MAR, Casis-Hao RJ, and Nano ALM Comparative effectiveness of probiotic strains on the prevention of pediatric atopic dermatitis: a systematic review and network meta-analysis Pediatr Allergy Immunol. 2021 Aug;32(6):1255–1270. doi: 10.1111/pai.13514. Epub 2021 May 15. PMID: 33811784. Cultrurelle Kids Daily Probiotic (chewable or packets) also has level I evidence and is available in Canada for childhood eczema and atopic dermatitis.

45 https://youtu.be/cgEbpNL9PSg

46 Turan B, Bengi G, Cehreli R, Akpınar H, Soytürk M. Clinical effectiveness of adding probiotics to a low FODMAP diet: a randomized, double-blind, placebo-controlled study World J Clin Cases. 2021 Sep 6;9(25):7417-7432. doi: 10.12998/wjcc.v9.i25.7417. PMID: 34616808; PMCID: PMC8464468.

47 Citation: Selvaraj SM, Wong SH, Ser H-L, et al. Role of a low-FODMAP diet and probiotics on the gut microbiome in Irritable Bowel Disease (IBS) Prog Microbes Mol Biol 2020; 3(1): a0000069. https://doi.org/10.3687/pmmb.a0000069)

48 https://pubmed.ncbi.nlm.nih.gov/36140990/#&gid=article-figures&pid=figure-1-uid-0

49 Daniel Merenstein et al. (2023) Emerging issues in probiotic safety: 2023 perspectives, Gut Microbes, 15:1, DOI: 10.1080/19490976.2023.2185034

50 https://isappscience.org/popular-media-misinformation-and-biotics/

51 https://internationalprobiotics.org/ipa-response-to-recent-washington-post-article/

52 Li H, He J, Jia W. The influence of gut microbiota on drug metabolism and toxicity. Expert Opin Drug Metab Toxicol. 2016;12(1):31-40. doi: 10.1517/17425255.2016.1121234. Epub 2015 Dec 10. PMID: 26569070; PMCID: PMC5683181

53 A systematic review and meta-analysis Sheyholislmai, H. et al., Nutrients, 2021 Jul; 13(7):2382